A Son's Journey

For Marcy & Bill,

That you may know our dear Jim, his goodness and courage, and our tremendous loss.

Dona Deininger

June 23, 2002

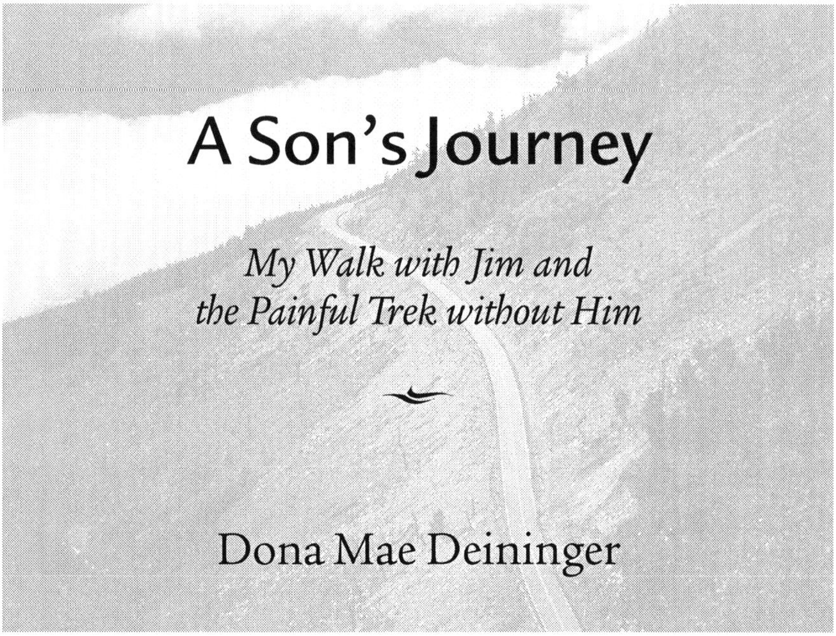

A Son's Journey

My Walk with Jim and the Painful Trek without Him

Dona Mae Deininger

White Pine Press

LCCN: 2001 132316
ISBN: 0-9710808-0-1

White Pine Press
Email: whitepinepress@qwest.net

Dustjacket and Interior design by Wendy Holdman
Typesetting by Stanton Publication Services, Inc.
Printing by Bookmobile, Inc.
Binding by Midwest Editions, Inc.

To the memory of our son,

James Jon Deininger

Jim gave so much to our lives,
and, in his suffering and death,
gave us the example and strength
to go on.

Table of Contents

Acknowledgments

I AM GRATEFUL TO MY HUSBAND, AL, FOR THE SUPPORT HE has given me in pursuing my idea for this book. Helpful, also, were the reading reviews and suggestions of Jim's sisters Kathy and Jeanne, and his brothers Bryan and Steve. They read my draft, gave me suggestions, and helped shape my in-process manuscript. Steve and Jeanne were nearby and available for technical support and she and Al assisted me in the final proofreadings.

Many friends and relatives, on hearing that I was writing a book about Jim, encouraged me in my efforts. During the periods in my writing venture, when I was not being very productive, I remembered their expressions of confidence and I thank them for their empowerment. I appreciate, also, the advice and direction which I received initially from Sid and Sue Jackson of "J" Press.

Next, I wish to thank Chris Reeves, who critiqued my manuscript, and Mary Ann Nord, who is a first-class editor. Mary Ann took this beginner's work and, with skill and warmth, fine-tuned it and made it stronger. Both she and Chris were very thoughtful of my feelings in this emotional writing venture. An author said of Jackie-O, "You expect love and encouragement from your editor." That certainly is what Mary Ann and Chris gave me.

Finally, I am most appreciative to have worked with Wendy Holdman of Stanton Publication Services. Wendy is a caring person and a thoughtful professional who read my emotions and pain and, as a graphic designer, worked to find appropriate text and graphic elements to reflect these and to help me create a meaningful legacy.

Preface

ON AUGUST 13, 1990, WE LOST OUR FIRST-BORN SON. This was the greatest tragedy of our lives—the one I will never be able to forget. Today when I think of it, even now as I write these memoirs, the keenness of our loss comes back to me as fresh and as terrible as it was that dark summer night. That loss brought an end to the happiness that had been ours for the thirty-two short years that we had Jim with us on this earth.

Whenever Jim came home, the house came alive. When he came into a room, the room lit up. The "quiet" is torture. A shining light has gone out in our life and we have a deep inner pain. In his company, we strutted a bit! We were a cheerful and vital family. It was a happy life until this tragedy struck.

A gifted, beautiful child, Jim loved living and he lived the life he had to its fullest. Though always gentle, he did everything with gusto. He was intelligent but always fun loving, industrious and lively, obedient and high-principled. I can honestly say he never needed reprimanding nor a "cross" word. He had an appetite for knowledge and a good heart. His talents and potentials should not have ended in such an early death.

On Thanksgiving Day, 1985, Jim was summoned from his peaceful pursuits to face his battle with Hodgkin's disease. After surgery and radiation he had three good years in his self-started dental practice. Just as he was in a position to enjoy an amenity or two, he had his first recurrence. He, and we, did everything possible to save that precious life. He lived and labored, confident of his strength, compassionate in his heart, and clear in his mind.

Writing this has been something I knew I must do—in loving memory of Jim and as a testimonial to his courage. We were so proud of him and of his accomplishment in his too-short life. He was so cheated and deserved so much more. Having achieved success he could have enjoyed the fruits of his labors—as well as having a social life and getting on with his plans for a big family. (As a child he always said he wanted twelve children but that may have changed a bit as he grew older.)

Filled with so much promise, blessed with every gift except length of years, what would this handsome young man be now, ten years later? A husband, father, and, yes, a caring, fun-loving son and brother, I think. I wish he could have known a wife and children and that Al and I could have known grandchildren from Jim. This remarkable young man with such high hopes for the future is in my thoughts each day. And, though ten years have passed, I still see a handsome, 32-year-old young man.

There have been times since Jim's death, especially when I hear of someone surviving Hodgkin's Disease or another cancer at a much later stage, that I wonder why Jim had to die. I wish he were still here, growing in years like his friends, knowing the joys they know.

We grieve differently and, as this writing is about dealing with the emptiness, I write, also, for Jim's father, Al; his sisters, Kathy and Jeanne; and his brothers, Bryan and Steve. All of our lives were changed by Jim's death; we have all lost a unique relationship. Our family is no longer complete. The circle was broken and the scale is no longer in balance. It is impossible to understand why this beautiful, special person has been taken from us so soon. His energy brought strength to our family.

No matter what activities and preoccupations there are, I can never forget the death of Jim. A great part of me died with Jim and I am not who I was. When a child's heart stops, so, in effect, does a parent's. As his mother, I have had to say good-bye to a part of myself. And the pain of that repeats itself both in my daily living and in each major event of life. The grief remains and I have only learned to live with it. Life does go on. It's horrible; but it does go on.

My pain has changed over ten years. At first, it seemed like a knife was being thrust into my chest and then turned. It hurt so I almost felt I could touch the pain. Now it is more a subdued, ever-present, numbing ache—a pervasive loneliness that comes from missing our son and from remembering his suffering and anguish.

Writing this book has helped me in knowing that I have done something that will help others know of Jim's courage and caring, his humbleness and greatness. It was written from my heart and it was written in pain. In my remembering, I hope those who knew Jim will do so, also.

If anyone should ever wonder about my innermost thoughts and feelings, they need only read *Lament for a Son* by Nicholas Wolterstorff, who lost a young son in a mountain climbing accident. His every thought is my thought; his every word is what I would say. He articulates in a manner I cannot. Reading it would enable one to see into my soul. He wrote:

> *Was he special? Did I love him more—more than his sisters and brothers? When they see my tears, do they think I loved him more?. . . . I love them equally though differently. . . . Each has an insight in which I delight. I celebrate them all and love them each. . . . When I give thanks, I mention all five; when I lament, I mention only him.*

Another book I found comforting, *A Grief Observed* by C. S. Lewis, echoes my thoughts of loss and grief. He says the depth of our sorrow is in direct proportion to the measure of joy we knew—the joy our loved one brought to our living. That joy was so immense; now, the grief is so intense. It's impossible to love someone and not be wounded by their absence.

On the day Jim died, and in the days immediately following, I looked at people going about their lives as usual and I wondered how this day could be normal. I thought, "Don't they know what has happened? Shouldn't everything have stopped when Jim's life did?" It seems unbelievable that life can or should go on—but I guess it must.

Nature-caused deaths are hard to understand. Having a child with a long-term illness, and being that child's primary caregiver, results in an unimaginable closeness—as love intensifies in a parent tending to a sick child. My closeness to Jim during his illness developed to such an extent that the person I came to know best and care about most was that struggling young man. Save actually having the disease, walking through it with your child gives one a pain and sorrow that becomes its own battle.

At the time of Jim's bone marrow transplant and my colon cancer surgery, we had both been given nearly the same prognosis. Jim's was a 50-percent chance for survival; mine was 40-45 percent. I find it hard to understand how my life was spared and Jim's life was not.

I'm one of those people who cry easily; I inherited this from my dad. Someone once said to us, after my tears came, "You've got to get over this and put it behind you." Though we do get on with our lives, we do not "get over it." Please know that when I speak of Jim, I need you to share my memories. Jim existed! Loss has no end. It is forever. Another person said, "It's o.k.; it'll be all right." Wrong! "It could not possibly be o.k. or all right." There are no answers and sometimes there are no words. In the absence of knowing what to say, a hug is a good substitute, a loving touch that reaches the soul and heals. I am reminded of my emotions at the time of Jim's viewing and funeral. What helped me were embracing hugs which were both supportive and comforting.

Not speaking of Jim denies he was a part of our lives for those thirty-two precious and gifted years. I want people to know that I appreciate their speaking of Jim. When people speak of Jim and my tears flow, perhaps they think, "Oh, no, now I've made her think of him." I would want people to know that I am thinking of him always and he is ever present—as are the tears that are merely surfacing. Jim was my soul mate.

I struggle to understand. I do not know why God allowed this to happen. I *did* pray long and I *did* pray hard for Jim's recovery. He had so much life left to live, so much left to give. I do know that my grief has left me with an even deeper love and appreciation for family and friends and it has given a greater depth to my compassion.

What we have experienced is not part of the natural order. The order of our being is reversed when our child precedes us in death. For in losing a child's future, we lose a part of ours. And the death of a child is the beginning of an unending journey. We cannot escape from our grief, we can only manage to accept and deal with Jim's absence. When your child dies, you lose a part of your flesh and blood. It's a bit like labor pains, except that these go on forever. Bereavement is a part of our love and it is a process that is continuing.

For a parent who has lost a child, the worst fear is that that child will be forgotten. Hearing Jim's name spoken, having him remembered in conversation, helps allay that fear. This is the greatest gift anyone can give us. To be remembered is to have lived! I want the world to know he lived. I pray my book will help keep Jim's memory, and all he stood for, alive.

A Son's Journey

"Happiness from Heaven"

"HAPPINESS FROM HEAVEN." THAT QUOTE FROM JIM'S birth announcement was indeed what we experienced when we welcomed our first-born son into the world. And he would continue to give us that happiness throughout his thirty-two years. I gave birth to Jim on Holy Saturday morning, April 5, 1958, at 3:27 A.M. He would be the middle of our five children.

Upon discharge from St. Mary's Hospital in Wausau, Wisconsin, Jim and I returned home to 1509 E. Brown St.—just eight blocks from the hospital. Jim was eight days old when he was baptized on April 13 in St. James Catholic Church. His godparents were his paternal grandfather, John Deininger, and his maternal grandmother's first cousin, once-removed, Bets Weisenberger Pflieger. Named James Jon, he soon was called Jimmy and, later, Jim.

At birth, Jim weighed the most of our children—8 lbs., 7½ oz.—and was twenty inches in length. He had Al's blue eyes but blonde hair. A few years later, on one of our visits to the hospital, the nurses

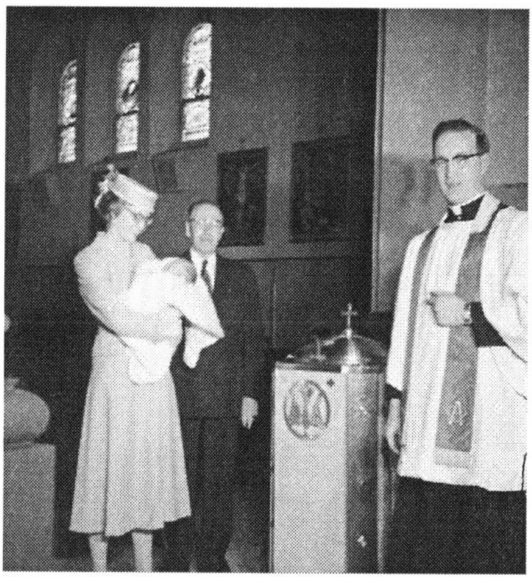

Jim's baptism with Godparents: Grandfather John Deininger and Cousin Bets Weisenberger Pflieger. Priest: Father Puerner

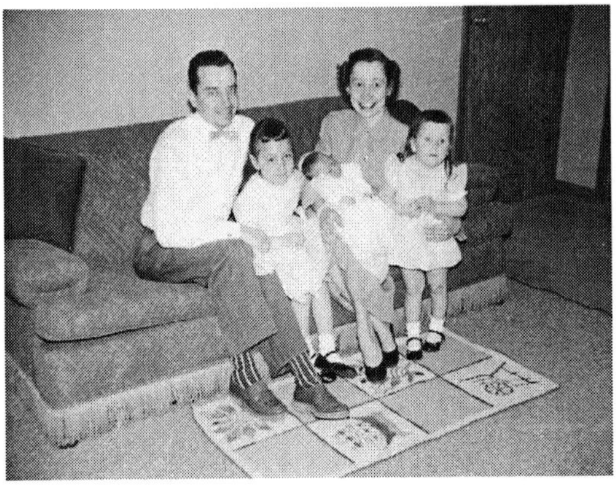

Our family of five at Jim's baptism, when he was one-week old

commented on how much he looked like Al. I remember being surprised by that—I guess because Al has such very dark hair. Many years later one of Jim's fellow dentists saw a picture of Al and me at the Omnitheatre—in a display of honeymooning couples at Niagara Falls. The dentist told Jim he had first thought it was a picture of Jim.

Jim always had a great appetite. To this day, I remember his record nursing—about every two hours, day and night, until he was six weeks old. He had a good head of hair and Al gave Jim his first haircut at eight months. Always a happy baby, he was a real joy for his father and me and for his two proud sisters, Kathy and Jeanne.

A Toddler in Wausau

JIM SPENT HIS FIRST SIX YEARS IN WAUSAU. THOUGH AS AN infant he had occasional bouts with croup and ear infections that necessitated several evening trips to the hospital, he was otherwise very healthy. As a toddler, and because of these infections, he had surgery for the removal of his tonsils and adenoids. In those years this surgery was often the recommended treatment.

One of our favorite stories of Jim as a toddler involved an incident, shortly after he learned how to talk, when he was helping

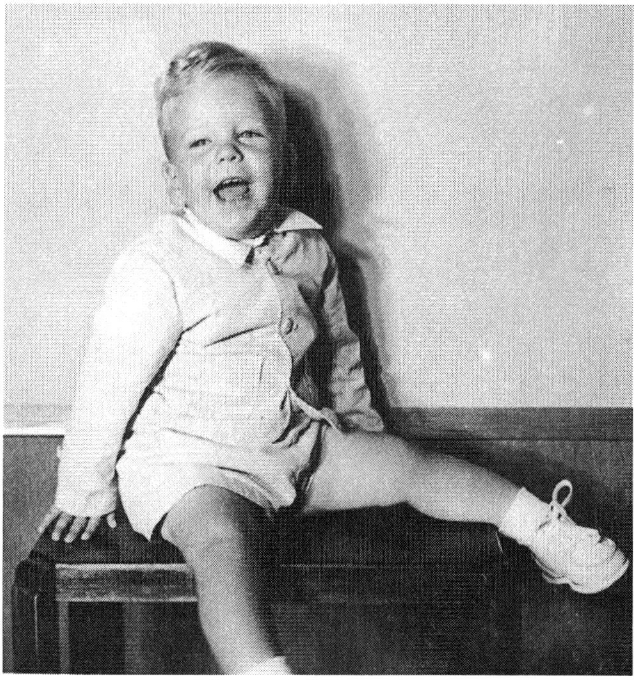

Jim at one year of age

Jim with Kathy and Jeanne at first-birthday party for twin cousins, Tracy and Anne, 1959

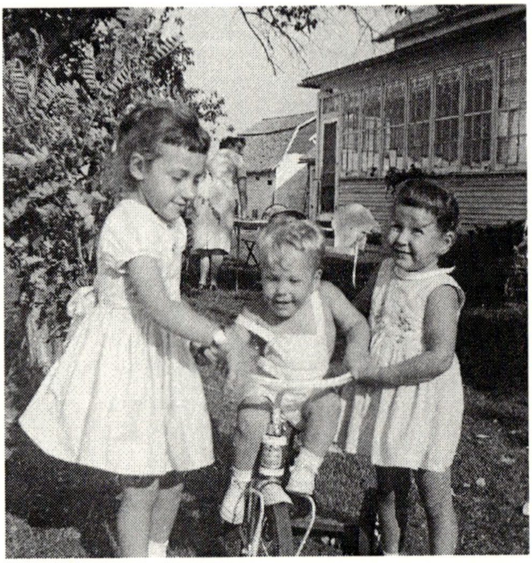

Al get the Christmas decorations from the attic. After being told not to touch the ornaments, Jim picked up one little wooden angel—and dropped it. He bent over to pick it up and said, "Ooh, me lucky this plastic!"

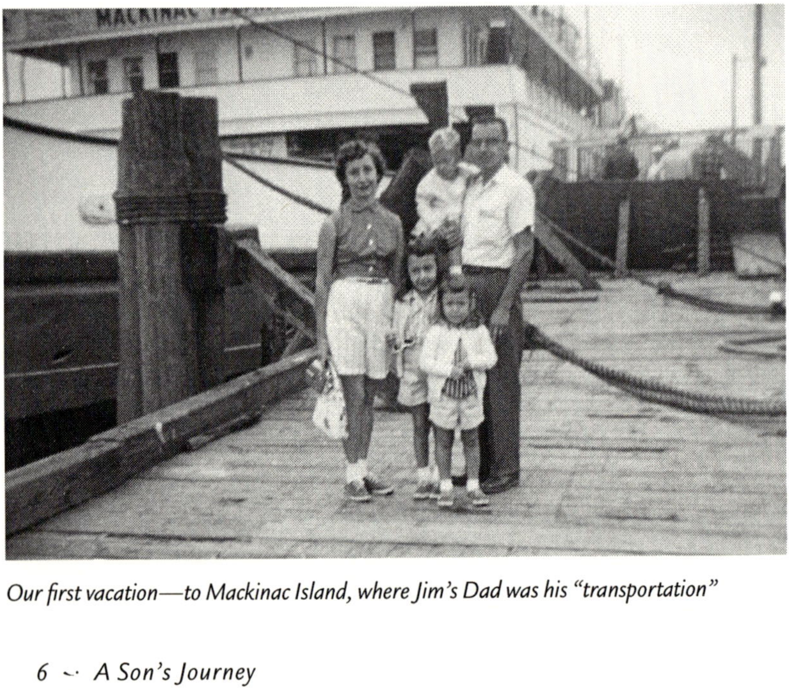

Our first vacation—to Mackinac Island, where Jim's Dad was his "transportation"

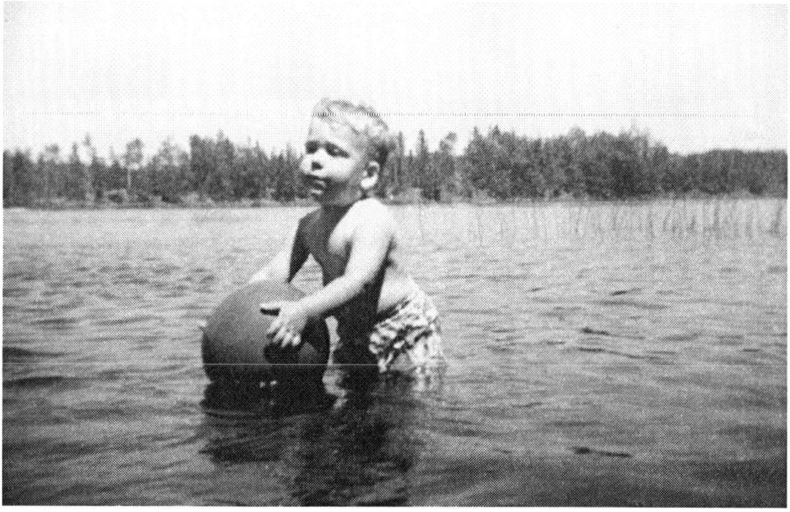

In the lake he came to love

Our family had a colonial rambler on ten acres of land just blocks outside the city limits. Jim's grandparents, my parents Agnes and August Kraimer, lived next door. His sisters were in school by the time brother Bryan was born, and so Bryan became Jim's playmate. He taught Bryan how to use the glider of the gym set, and they had their own little vegetable gardens.

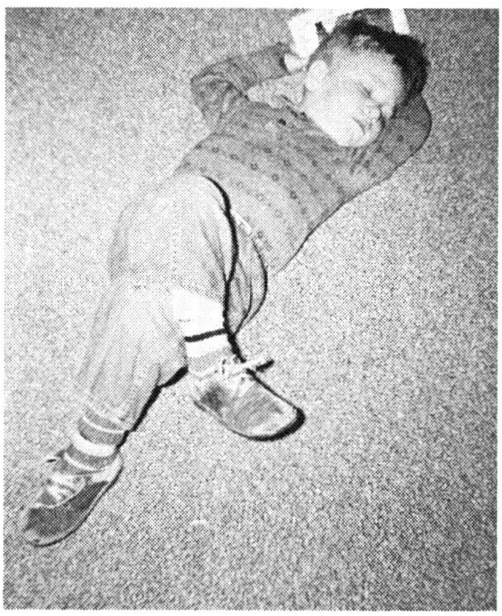

"Nodding off" with a good book

Jim was always a real "ham." Once I noticed he had put up a chaise lounge right next to that of our neighbor, Gladys Schaible, so that he too could soak up some sun. Gladys and Bob gave Jim his first nickname, "Jimbo." They also gave the children their first pets—colored chicks for Easter.

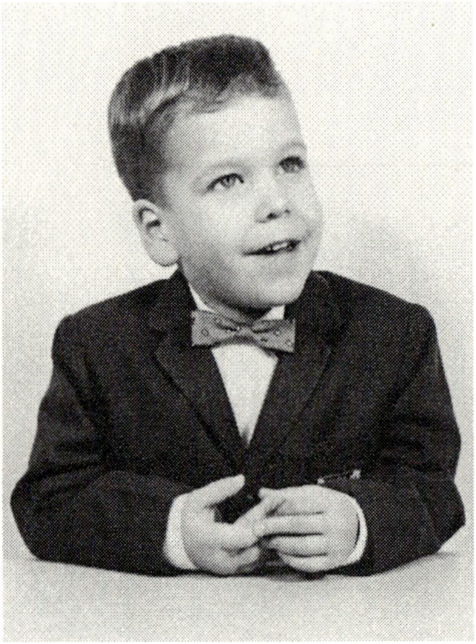

A gentleman at age two-and-one-half years

We spent a good share of our summer weekends at my parents' cottage in Tomahawk, Wisconsin. One summer on our first trip of the year to the cottage, Jim jumped from the car and ran to the hill that sloped down to the lake. Gathering momentum down the hill and unable to stop, he ran straight into the lake! With the presence of mind Jim always had, he just stood up and walked back out.

Attending the county fairs each summer was another highlight for the children. For about three years we had four white rabbits, and the children had leashes for them. In the winter, we ice-skated as a family, and Jim would ski and sled with us on the hill behind our home.

At age five Jim went off to Wausau Senior High School—that is, to a kindergarten in the building. Even back then, Jim was the scholar—going to high school at age five. Jim's two older sisters had done the same. During that school year, when I was pregnant with Steve, we decided to tell the children the news at bedtime. As we were kneeling for prayers alongside the

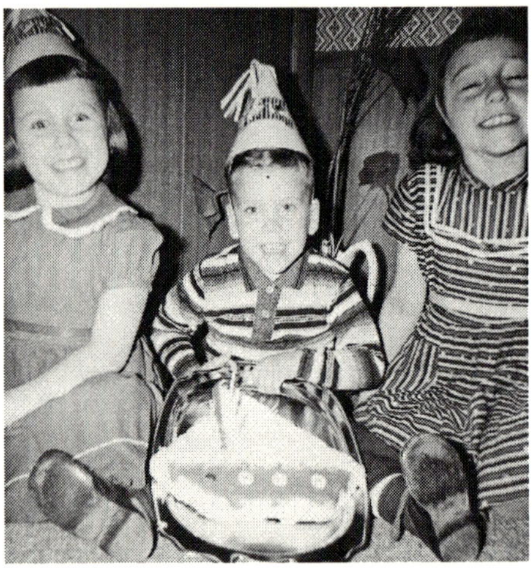

Jim's third birthday—with sisters Kathy and Jeanne and Mom's "boat cake"

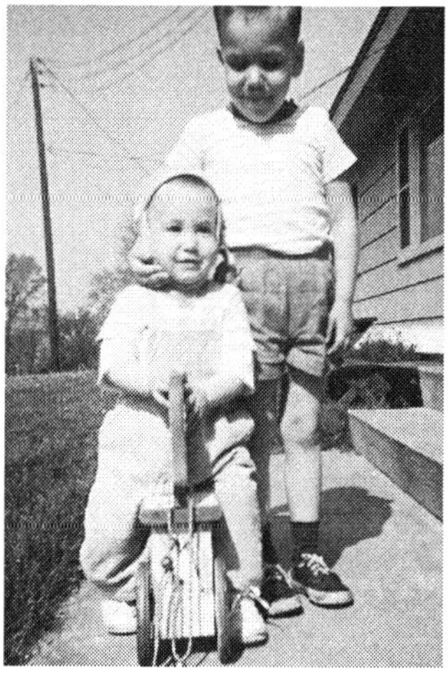

With his brother, Bryan . . .

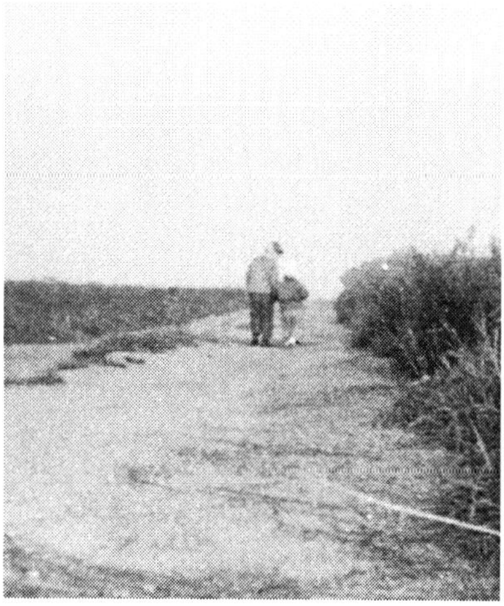

walking the "back ten"

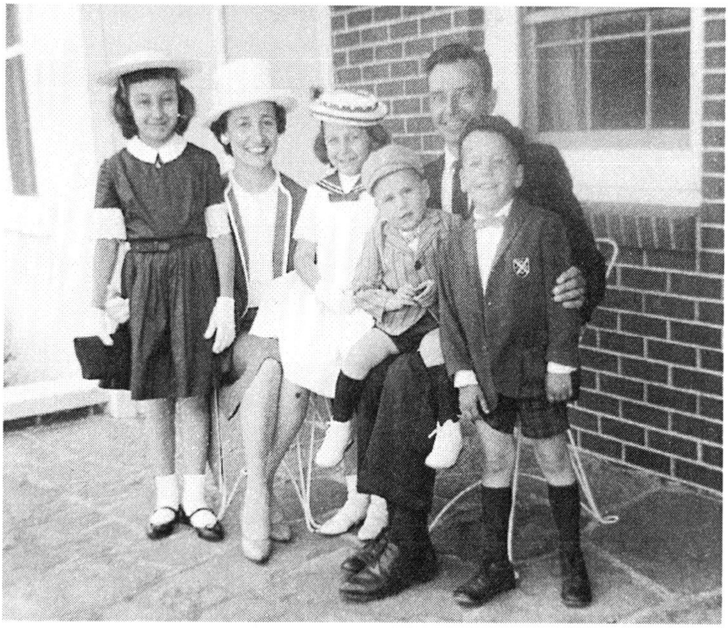

Mothers' Day, 1963

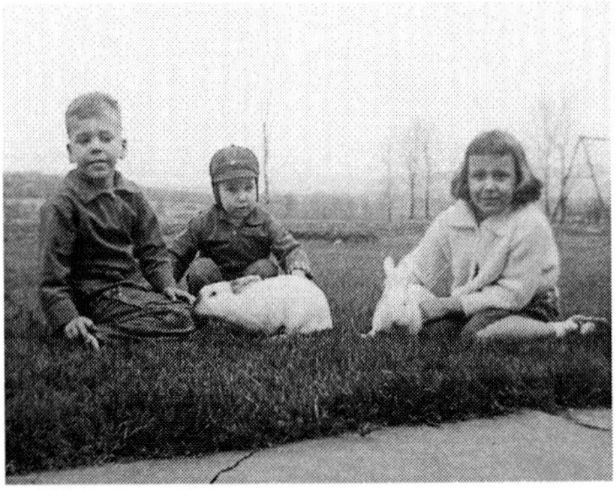

Jim, Bryan and Jeanne with two of our four white rabbits

bed, we did so. Jim said, "I'm so happy." We answered, "Yes, so are we"—to which Jim added, "Now I have something for 'show and tell' tomorrow."

In the summer of 1964, when I was eight months pregnant with Steve, Al accepted a position with Skelly Oil Company and we awaited Steve's birth and our subsequent move to Madison, Wisconsin. Years later Jim recounted several times how eager he was to see the new baby when Mother returned home from the hospital. He said he looked him over well, noticing the little fingers and toes, and thinking this might be the last baby "we" would have. After Steve's birth, we prepared for our move.

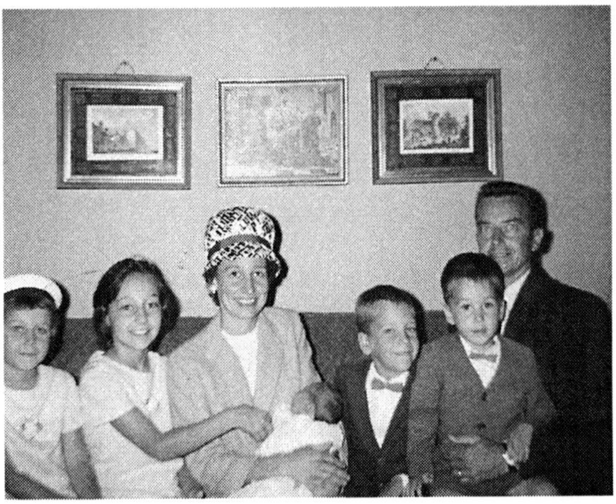

Our family of seven, with six-day-old brother Steven, on his day of baptism (Aug. 9, 1964)—five weeks before we moved to Madison, Wisconsin

Madison Happy Days

Our family of seven moved to Madison when Steve was one month old. The nine and one-half years we would spend in this beautiful, friendly city would be some of the happiest and most carefree years of our lives. We lived in a lovely two-story colonial on Woods End, a cul-de-sac of fifteen homes and about fifty children. Jim entered first grade at Our Lady Queen of Peace Elementary School. The children could now walk a couple of blocks to school and could come home for lunch. It was an exciting and different lifestyle for us. We had oak trees and

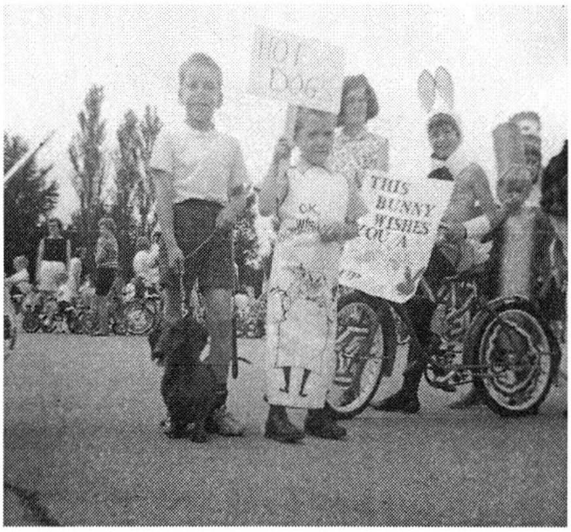

Jim and Bryan with their "hot-dog" Hans in the Fourth of July parade. They were unable to keep Hans within the hot dog bun they'd made.

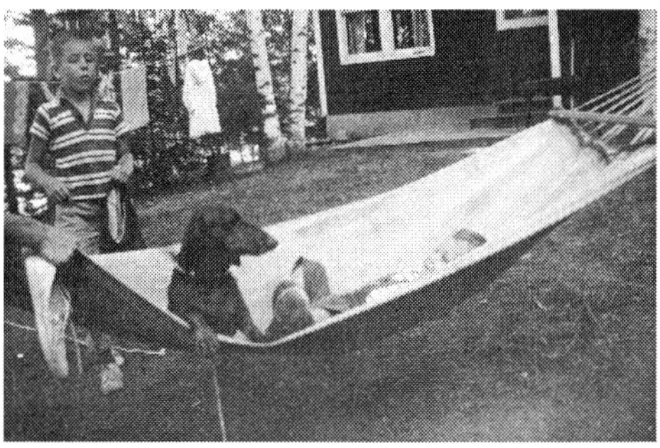

Jim pushing the cottage hammock to give Steve and Hans a ride

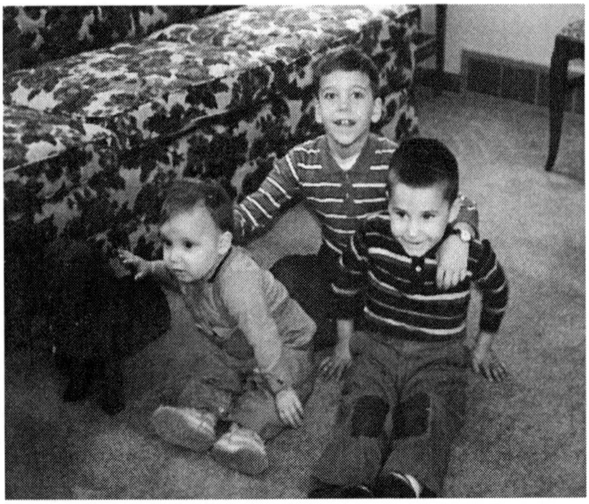

Jim, Bryan and Steve with Hans, our dachshund

plenty of leaves for raking in the fall. Neighborhood children clamored to get into our fenced yard! Halloween meant the children could "trick-or-treat" at some fifty homes without crossing a street—as the area included two cul-de-sacs. And then, our new neighbors, the Dischs, gave us our first dog. Hans, a dachshund, would be ours for about nine years.

The transition to life in Madison was easy. Though the children missed not being near their grandparents, we visited them

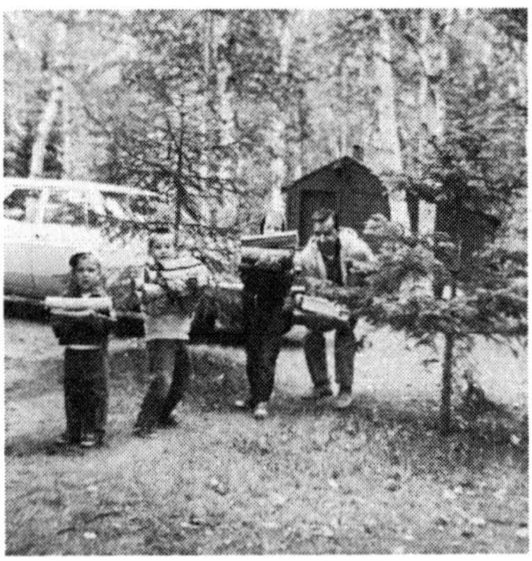

Bringing in the wood: Steve, Bryan and Jim with Dad

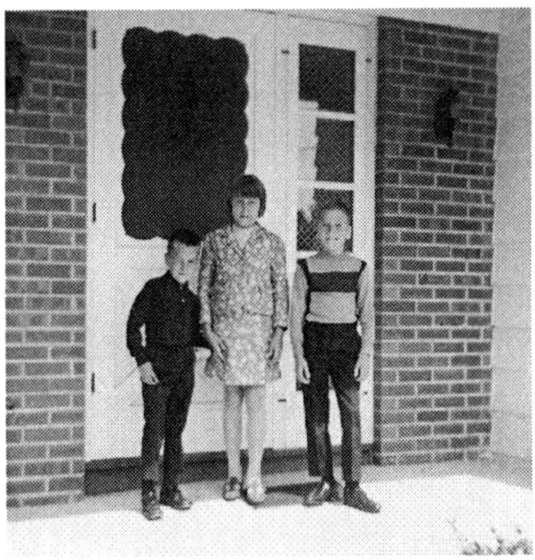

Back to school, 1967: Bryan, Jeanne, Jim

often. And, we had much company: grandparents from Wausau, as well as other out-of-town relatives and friends. In the winter, we went north for the children to enjoy time snowmobiling with their grandparents—a sport their grandparents did well into their eighties. In the summer, we continued to travel to the cottage for weekends and vacations. And when Jim was about nine years old, he learned how to water-ski. Then in 1970, we got our first speedboat—at Christmas time. Had people been able to peer into our garage, they would have wondered about us. The children were so excited, they couldn't wait for summer and so they could be found sitting in the boat, in the garage, in winter, listening to their new eight-track tapes.

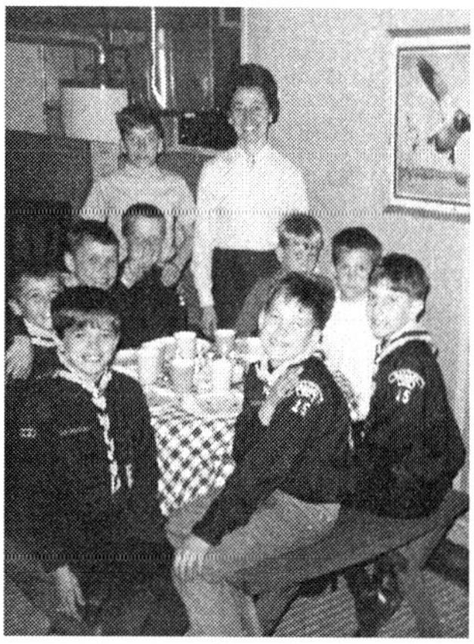

Den Chief Jim helping Den Mother Dona in Bryan's Cub Scout Pack

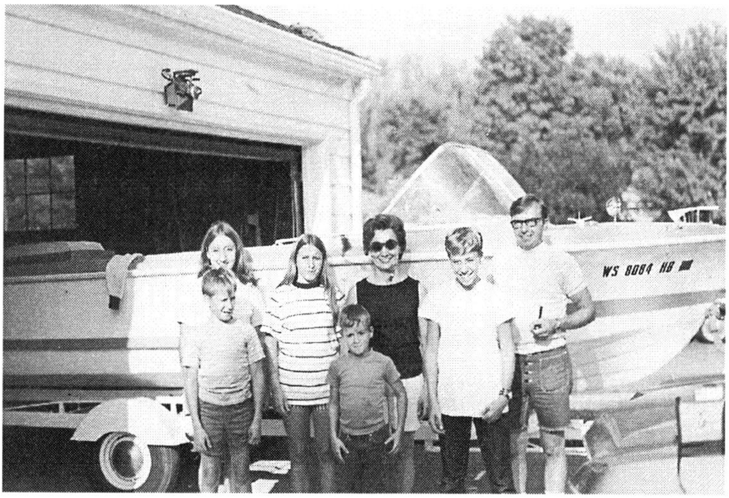

Our family with our first speedboat, 1971

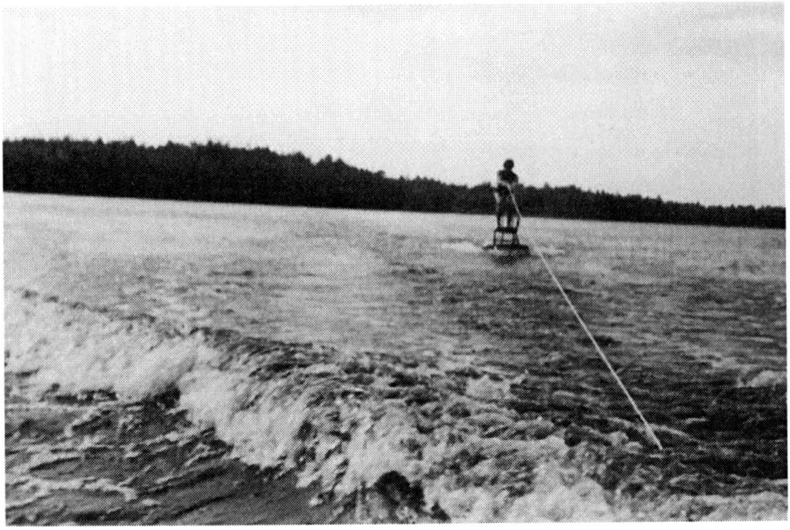

Jim water-skiing (on a chair, on a saucer), 1972

Water-skiing was a sport at which Jim would become proficient, as would Bryan and Steve. In fact, we all became water skiers. There were times when Al would pull up to eight skiers at a time. Jim was soon making turns on a saucer—then standing on a chair he put on top of the saucer. I remember his attempts to ski barefoot and make starts from the dock. When we later moved to Minnesota, Jim and Bryan would learn to ski off a jump. The boys would motivate me, too, and that is perhaps how I began to ski slalom. One experience really stands out—when the boys talked me into trying their new graphite ski. It was a thrilling adventure; I had only to *think* of turning or to glance in another direction and I went. I was never so happy to see shore!

In grade school, Jim also learned to swim and progressed through lifesaving classes. Swimming, too, would become a lifelong sport for him. I know there were many times, when he was a student at the University of Minnesota, he would go to Bierman Hall and swim for relaxation.

Jim was active in both Cub Scouts and Boy Scouts. I was den mother for our three sons' packs and Al was assistant scoutmaster for the troop. Jim went to Scout camp each summer and we were so proud of him, when, in 1972, he was inducted into the Order of the Arrow, which is a thing of the spirit. The order recognizes the qualities of brotherhood, cheerfulness, and service. He was elected to the order by his fellow Scout campers, who saw those traits in him. After the Ordeal–a 24-hour outdoor journey to test those strengths–he was welcomed into the order in a Brotherhood ceremony.

In Madison Jim got his first job–a big step in his maturing and another example of his industriousness and business acumen. Without our knowing it, he had, for about a year, been badgering one of the Madison newspapers for a route as a carrier. On his twelfth birthday, the route supervisor called to say they had a route for him. He was a newspaper carrier for three years, had his own checking account at age twelve and saved every cent he earned. The paper route had been serviced with a used $10, double-rear-basketed bike. (When he was much younger, his first new bike had been a sporty "banana seat". Some years earlier this had been stolen when he biked to the local hobby shop to buy a birthday gift for his brother–the one time the bike wasn't locked.)

Jim served his customers well. He always placed their papers between the doors and when he would be gone for a weekend he left notes with the name and phone number of his substitute carrier. His monthly collection trip took several hours because he included visiting time with the elderly on his route, even sitting with them to look through their photo albums when he sensed they needed company. We were astounded when his first Christmas as a carrier produced $90 in tips (this was 1970!), as well as gifts of homemade cookies and candy. One day he brought home an injured bird he had found and, after nursing it back to health, was able to happily release it. His sister, Kathy, remembers the time when, during a heavy rain, with his jacket hood pulled down, he ran into a parked car, bending the handlebars of his bike. When he finished three years as a news carrier he had saved $1,500 and bought for himself a new Schwinn bike.

Coordinating the many activities and schedules of Jim and his four siblings was possible because of the convenient location of our home on the west side of Madison. Though Al was on the road a great deal, and we were a one-car family for most of our years in Madison, we did manage. I would try to schedule the children for dental checkups to follow each other. At the end of the day, our neighbor-dentist, Dr. Bill Evans, would bring the children home with him. We would usually bike several miles for our doctor appointments at Dean Clinic and, also, bike to the Swim Club, which was just a couple of miles from our home.

In His Own Words

WHEN JIM WAS IN SEVENTH GRADE ONE OF HIS ASSIGNMENTS was to write an autobiography. As a supplement to this chapter in his life, I add this work. These were his own thoughts and words. My only help was in typing the assignment.

My Autobiography

By Jim Deininger

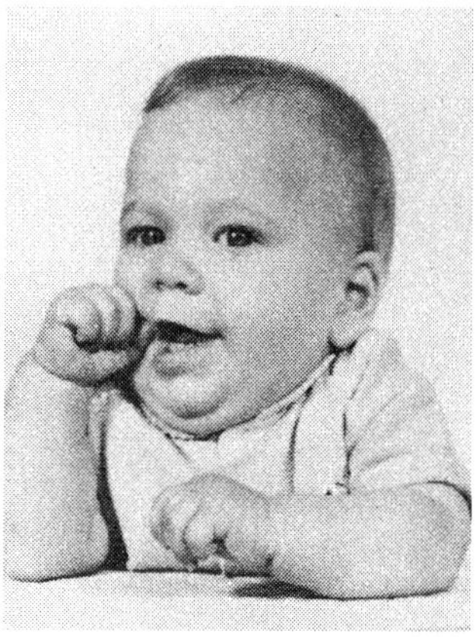

Most babies are brought by a stork but I was brought by the Easter Bunny. For I was born on Easter Eve. This historical happening took place in Wausau, Wisconsin—about 140 miles from Madison—in St. Mary's Hospital on April 5, 1958. The lucky parents are Dona and Alwin Deininger. I was their first son and am now the middle of five children. I got my brown hair from Mom, my blue eyes from my Dad, and my baby shoes from my sister—who got them handed down from my oldest sister. But we are still trying to find out who I got my mouth from. Most people say that it looks like my Mom's and Dad's put together.

When I was a year old I went on my first long trip to Mackinac Island, Michigan. There were no vehicles allowed on the island, but I didn't find transportation hard—mainly because my Father carried me.

Two years after the Easter Bunny brought me, he brought three, colored baby chicks for my two sisters and me. Mine was blue and we named him Doc. It was a real surprise he lived—mainly because I didn't treat him too gently.

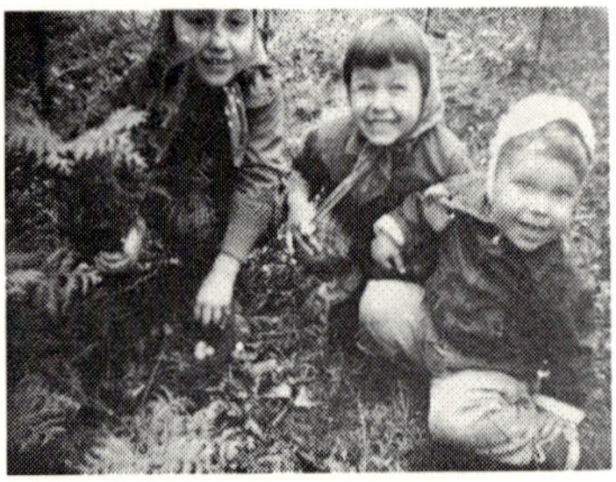

My grandparents, Mr. and Mrs. August Kraimer have a cottage in Tomahawk, Wisconsin, and for miles they are surrounded by woods. When I was two years old my sisters, Kathy who was seven and Jeanne who was five, went exploring with me and guess what we found—a bird nest with three eggs in it.

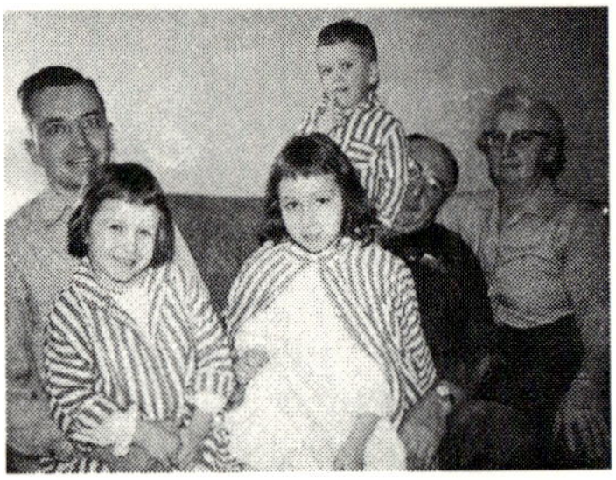

When I was two and one half years old, I would hate to go to bed. Right before bedtime I would try to think of some way I could stay up a bit longer. When this picture was taken, you can tell that I am in great thought.

When I turned three I had a wonderful birthday. My Mom baked me a delicious cake in the shape of a boat.

During this same year our family was evened off. We then had two girls and two boys. We named my brother Bryan.

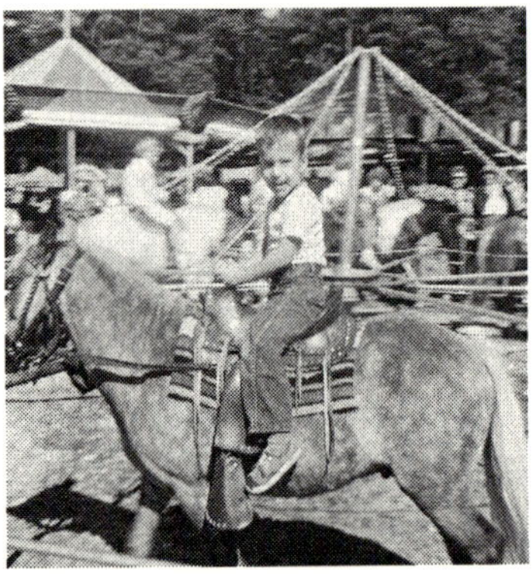

Every year in Wausau, there was a fair. When I was younger I went on, mostly, the merry-go-round; but the year I was four, I headed straight for the horses. I got on and, boy, did I go; I feel if I would have let go this would be the end of my autobiography. I still look forward to the fair every year and try not to miss it.

When I was five, I took those first steps to school. My teacher's name was Miss Cawley, and her assistant, Miss Alice. One of the assignments that Miss Cawley gave us was to count, read, and write our numbers one through ten. That night I went home and, mis-

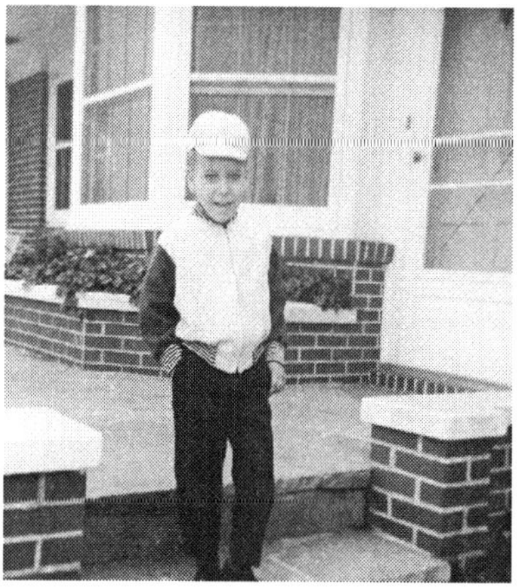

takenly, told my Mom that I had to learn one through 100. By 10:00 P.M. I had learned to count, read, and write to 100. Even now I like going to school and coming home, but it's the time in between that that gets me.

I started off to school at Wausau Senior High—kindergarten. Every year at Wausau Senior High, they had a salt water taffy sale. Both my older sisters, Kathy and Jeanne, won by selling the most candy. Kathy won a large book of fairy tales called Mostly Magic; *and Jeanne also won a book of fairy tales, called* Stories That Never Grow Old. *They both still have these books. I came very close to selling the most, but I didn't quite make the top prize.*

The next summer we moved to Madison. I had a little going-away party with two of my friends—Fred Hirn and Ken Krieg. We hiked to a nearby park and ate our lunch. On the way we carried our lunches in a big red handkerchief, at the end of a pole which we put over our backs.

Five weeks before we moved we received a new member in our family and decided to name him Steven. We moved the day before school began. Kathy was eleven; Jeanne was nine; I was six; Bryan was three; and Steven was one month and eleven days. It was a sunny day, September 14. The people were still living in the house we bought, so we lived in a motel for four days. When we moved into the house we bought, there was a lot of unpacking to do. Our house is a two-story of mostly wood, with a brick front.

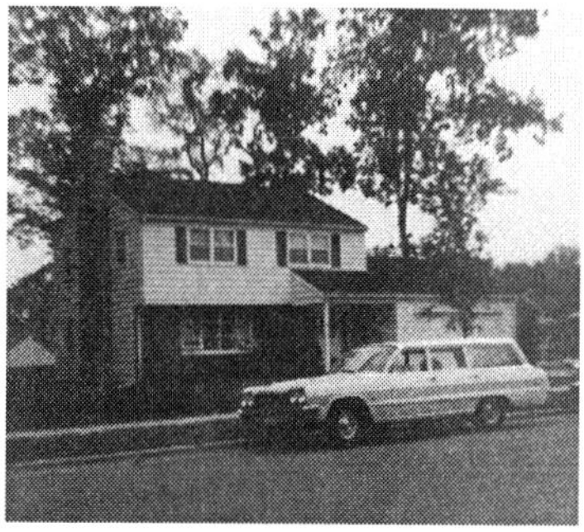

I entered the first grade with Mrs. Hamilton as my teacher. Near the end of the school year, Mrs. Hamilton planned a first-grade school play. I got the part of Humpty-Dumpty. No wonder everyone said I was cracking up!

After first grade, it wasn't long before we got a dog who was already named Hans. Our dog came with a few tricks. For one, he can hold a piece of bread on his nose until you say o.k. He can dance and jump through a hoop. Just recently he had a romance with a large female Saint Bernard. I'd better explain that Hans is a Dachshund.

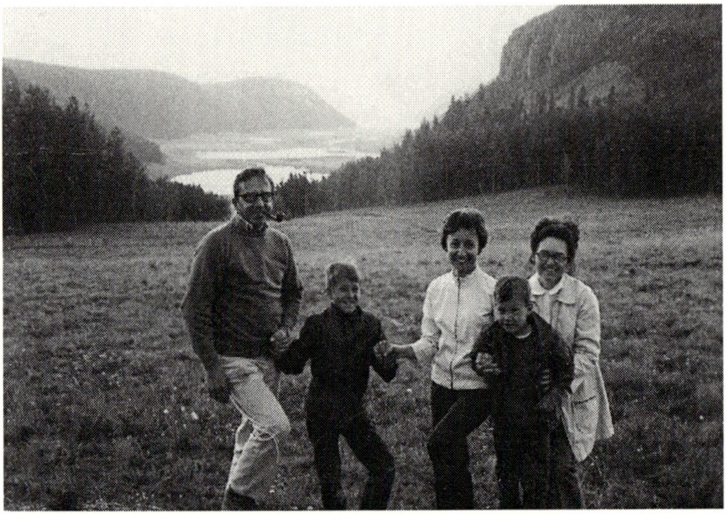

In the summer of my seventh year, our family visited our Aunt, Uncle, and six cousins in Colorado. We visited Canon City and Royal Gorge—which has the highest suspension bridge in the world. While we were there we rode the incline railway to the bottom of the Gorge. We visited Monarch Pass through the Continental Divide and went up a small trail to 12,000 feet. The sun had been shining below, but it was snowing up there.

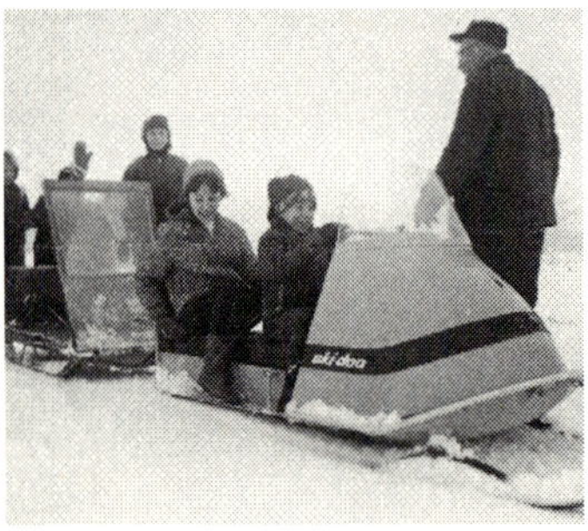

The next winter when I was seven, I drove my grandparents' snowmobile myself for the first time. Boy, was that fun.

That year on Mother's Day, 1966, I received my first Holy Communion at the 12:30 Mass at Our Lady Queen of Peace. Afterward, we had a big reception and dinner at home for my grandparents, godparents and friends.

During the school year I also started Cub Scouts, and, in May of 1967 we went on a father-son campout at Camp Grey.

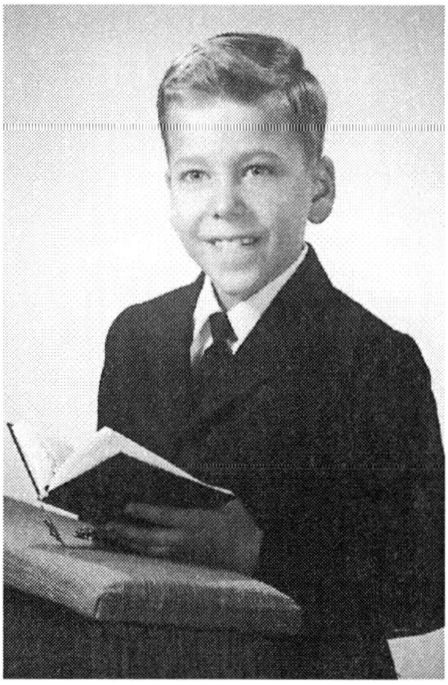

Every summer each child in our family spends a week or two alone with my grandparents at their home in Wausau. The summer I was nine, I went on my first ride on a jet—to Madison from Wausau. When I boarded the plane at Wausau, the first stop was Stevens Point, where quite a few people got on. Someone sat down next to me, and we talked. When we got to Madison I almost forgot to get off. But the man next to me told me, and they opened the doors for me. That summer I also got up on water skis and, boy, was that fun!

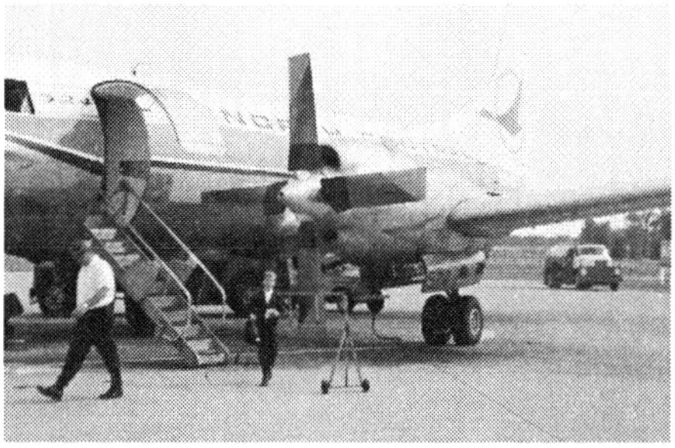

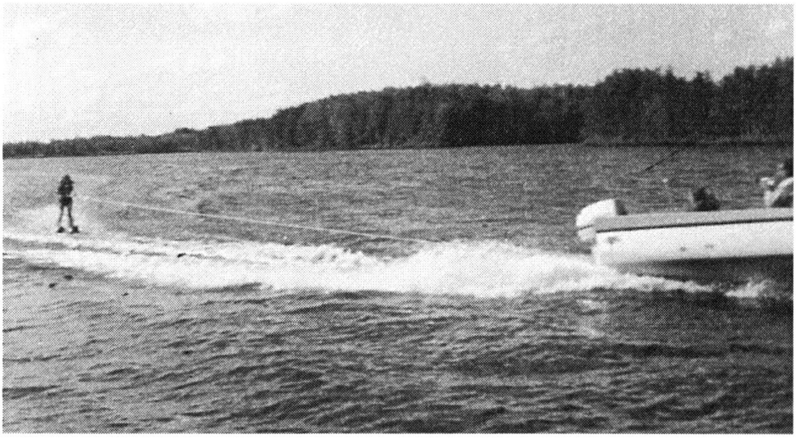

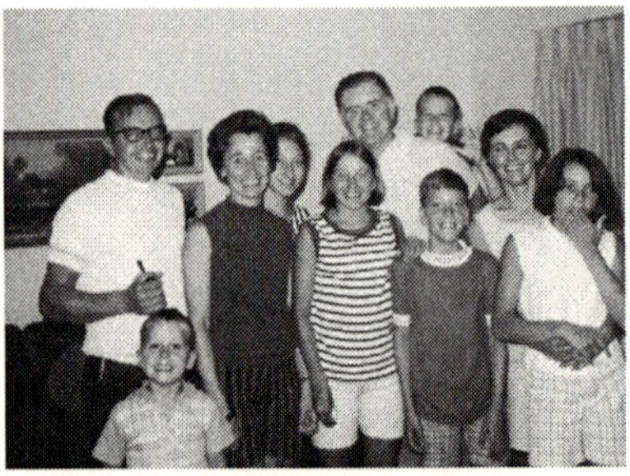

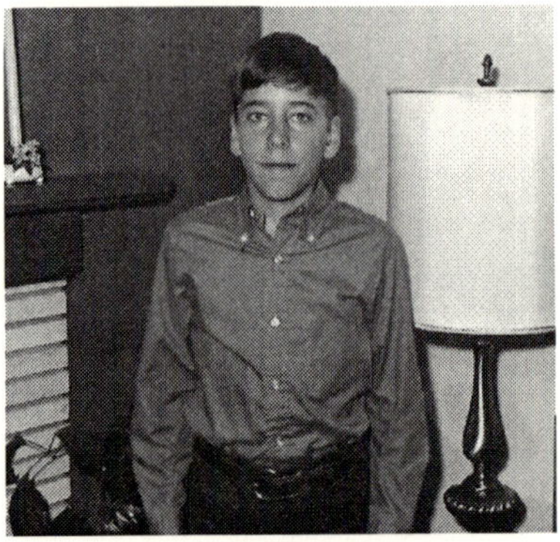

In fourth grade we had a lot of fun; and, for our field trip, we went to Little Norway and Cave of the Mounds. I liked Little Norway better. I also took piano lessons this year and in the summer following.

When I was eleven, our family and my grandparents—nine of us—went by station wagon on a trip to New Jersey and Washington, D.C. In New Jersey, we visited one of Dad's Navy buddies, whom he hadn't seen in twenty years. There we swam in the Atlantic Ocean at Ship Bottom, where the waves are about fifteen feet high. In Washington we visited the White House; had lunch in the Old Senate Office Building; saw the Capitol, National Archives, Smithsonian Museum of History and Technology, National Shrine of the Immaculate Conception, Georgetown, and the Lincoln, Washington, and Jefferson Memorials. We also visited Mount Vernon; Arlington National Cemetery; and had a private tour of the Pentagon, by one of Secretary Mel Laird's assistants.

I went on to Boy Scouts in the fifth grade and we have a campout one weekend each month; my favorite was Eagle Cave. Also in the fifth grade, I took guitar lessons and enjoy playing the guitar. In April I got my paper route and still have it. I have 62 customers and delivering and collecting take up a lot of my time. This last summer I went to Boy Scout Camp for a week at Camp Castle Rock; and, like every other summer, went to my grandparents' home and cottage. I also enjoy swimming in the summer at West Side Businessmen's Club.

I have had the very nicest teachers at Queen of Peace School. After Miss Hamilton, I've had Sister Carlo, Mrs. Whittington, Mrs. Murphy, Mrs. Keyser, Mrs. Rengstorff, Mrs. Nord; and now, Sister Viola and Mrs. Rosario. I like it here!

As he expressed, Jim's years at Our Lady Queen of Peace were very happy ones: his first crush, a myriad of friends, progressive teaching nuns, and happy Scout days. Then, one year later, when Jim was in the eighth grade, Al received a promotion. This meant we would be leaving Madison for the Twin Cities.

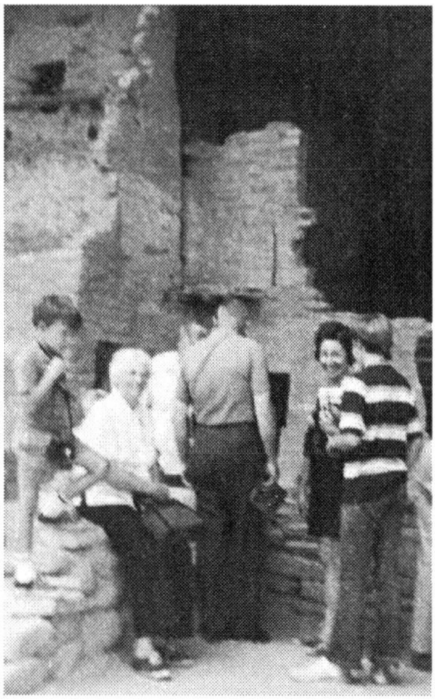

Mesa Verde, 1972—Steve, Grandparents Kraimer, Mom and Jim

Jim's coed going-away party for eighth-grade friends was at our home and included dancing. It also included a chipped front tooth, which was smoothed down by Dr. Bill. Did Jim's exposure to the life of a dentist lead to Jim's decision to become a dentist? Al and I had always thought this child—a great communicator, with the ability to talk and command an audience—would perhaps be a priest or an attorney. I guess a career as a dentist wasn't too far-fetched; Jim still had a captive, quiet audience.

Days in Dellwood

IT WAS A SAD DAY FOR JIM AND HIS BROTHERS, AS WELL AS Mom, when we had to leave Madison in January of 1973 to move to Minnesota. (Dad was happy!) Jim's two sisters stayed in Madison. Kathy was at the University of Wisconsin and Jeanne, a senior at Edgewood High School, lived with our very dear friends, Joan and Ron Janssen and family, while she completed her senior year at Edgewood.

As we drove into our new neighborhood, we stopped at the row of mailboxes and found in ours, an envelope from Kathy. In it was a poem she had sent to help lift our spirits. It expressed the fact that tomorrow does not automatically dawn a bright and sunny day. It is a process that requires hours of joys and sorrows. It made us realize, in our sadness, that we would have to work to create new memories for our happiness. Then, this dejected group sat down to a dinner which friends from Madison had sent in a basket–tablecloth, spaghetti, bread sticks, and wine.

Before we even left Madison, Bryan wasn't feeling well, and on our first night in our new home, all three boys were sick. We had moved at the end of the semester, and Jim had to leave eighth grade, mid-year. His brothers were in fifth and second grades. We lived in a more rural area and, though we had neighbors on multi-acre type lots, none of the area children went to the parochial school where our boys were registered. The school was very small and not at all as progressive as were our schools in Madison. The boys were unhappy and, therefore, so was Mom. In the morning, waiting for the bus, we had a "together time", when I read *The Swiss Family Robinson* to them. It was probably during this difficult time of adjustment that Jim began looking forward to driver's education as a way out of our newly isolated existence. On his desk, he kept a notepad that was headed, "Days till I can drive." It took several pages to cover these numbers of 699 to 0 and the countdown was marked with slashes—something Kathy had done, also.

We moved to Dellwood with our second dog, Patches. Patches had joined our family unplanned. When our children went with their grandparents to the family cottage in Tomahawk the previous year, they had stopped at the local supermarket. While their grandmother was in the store shopping, they saw a box marked "Free Puppies" and their grandfather had allowed them to choose one. By the time they had resumed their trip and their grandmother heard the puppy, it was too late.

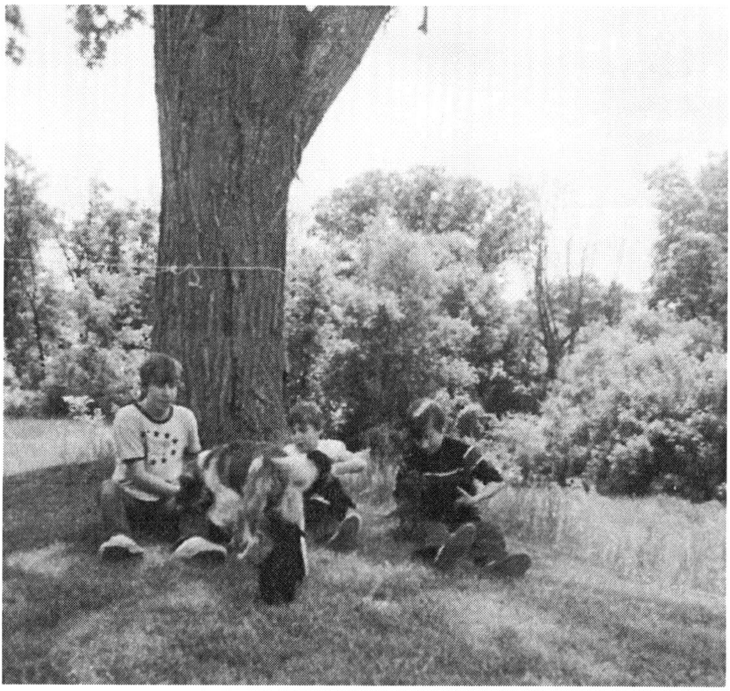

Jim, Steve and Bryan with Patches and some of her puppies

This sheltie-sized dog, the vet believed, was crossbred of collie and German shepherd. She was mild-mannered and very intelligent. Some months after we'd moved, we realized Patches was going to have a litter. As the time for delivery approached, we readied a "birthing place" and took her temperature daily. The principal of the boys' school had said they could be dismissed when Patches began having the puppies. So, when the time arrived, I picked up the boys from school and they were able to witness the birth of the seven puppies. Jim had told us that on the day of delivery, the dog-dad should make an appearance. Sure enough, on the day Patches delivered her puppies, a black lab from several blocks away spent the day outside our garage door! This whole episode gave us some welcome excitement. And we have movies of the black lab playing with the puppies weeks later on our front lawn. As we found homes for the puppies, Jim had me keep a list of the names and addresses of the owners so that one day, when he was older, he might have one of Patches' puppies. Al, Jim, and our other children trained her well. She was a gentle, intelligent dog.

One neighbor family, the Smiths, had boys the same age as Jim and Bryan. They were especially friendly and helpful to us in our new locale. Jim's sisters visited often and brought their brothers' friends to visit. At the end of the school year, eighth-grader Jim was invited back to graduate with his class at Queen of Peace in Madison. The following year, he went to Hill-Murray High School, a parochial school about ten miles from our home. Jim was a model student who filled his day with as many classes as he could—claiming he might as well get as much as he could for the tuition. Jim and his four brothers and sisters, through all of their high school and college years, paid for half of their tuition themselves—though Jim insisted on covering his full college tuition, while we paid half of his fraternity dues and housing.

Jim had two jobs in high school. He worked first at a Country Kitchen restaurant, starting with loading the dishwasher. He was soon assisting the cook—experience that proved useful later when he had his own home and would enjoy cooking. One morning at 2:00 A.M. as he was driving home from the late shift, his car was broadsided by another on the highway. Though the car was "totaled" by the insurance company, Jim escaped without a scratch. (Everyone always considered Jim to be lucky.)

In his next job, at Powers Department Store, Jim worked as a salesperson in the men's clothing department. There he learned about fine clothing and colors and was able, at a discount, to accumulate a nice wardrobe. He continued to work at Powers into his college years.

Sometime during his high school years Jim began volunteering at the Red Cross. He began donating blood and would continue to do so until his diagnosis. I recall one Christmas Eve day, when all of the family was together, Jim suggested his siblings join him when he went down to the Red Cross to donate blood. They did and he said, "Now we've given our holiday gift for those in need." Later, in college, he resumed volunteering at the Red Cross. Qualified to teach CPR classes, one Thanksgiving weekend at the cottage he gave all of us gathered the CPR course.

Jim's years at Hill-Murray High School were to net him tried-and-true friends. (From high school into his dental practice

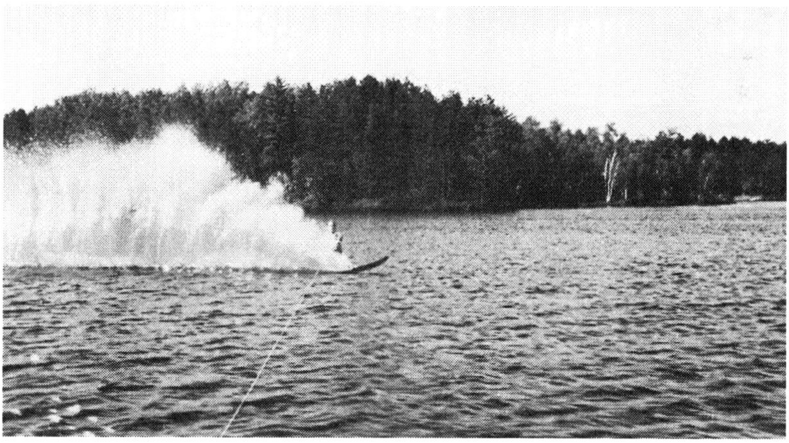

Jim, skiing slalom

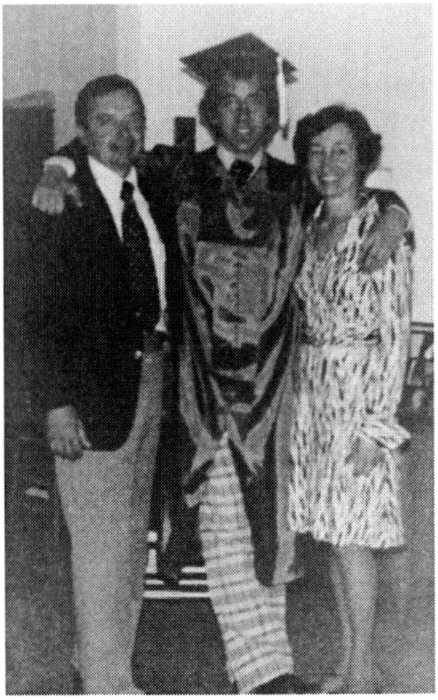

A carefree Jim with Mom and Dad on his graduation from Hill-Murray High School, 1977

venture, from his diagnosis to his death, they were exemplary. They, and their wives, were for Jim, and still are for us, one of our strong support groups.) Jim sang in the choir in high school. He was a good student but he hated wearing the required uniform. If a student came to school without the required tie, he had to go to the office to rent one for the day. It wasn't long before Jim probably owned one of the rented ties and just kept it in the office for storage. Jeanne remembers that when Jim graduated from Hill-Murray, he said he never wanted to wear a light-blue dress shirt again. And I know he never wanted to own another pair of black, smooth-toe oxford shoes.

I remember his many downhill skiing trips with Dave Paddock and the Ski Club and his frequent jogging around Lake Phalen with Rick Marty. Jim's friend, Mike Rieschl, remembers their days in art class. We have, among our treasures, much of his art-class work. This includes paintings, pottery and woodcarving.

Jim always shared so much with me: the books he read, the fun experiences he had. I especially remember Jim sharing with me an account of one of his evenings out. When he and his friends stopped at a stoplight, they noticed a group of young kids standing on the corner, smoking cigarettes. Jim and his friends rolled down the car windows and admonished the kids about the dangers of smoking. By the time the light turned to green, the smokers had thrown down their cigarettes and stomped them out. To

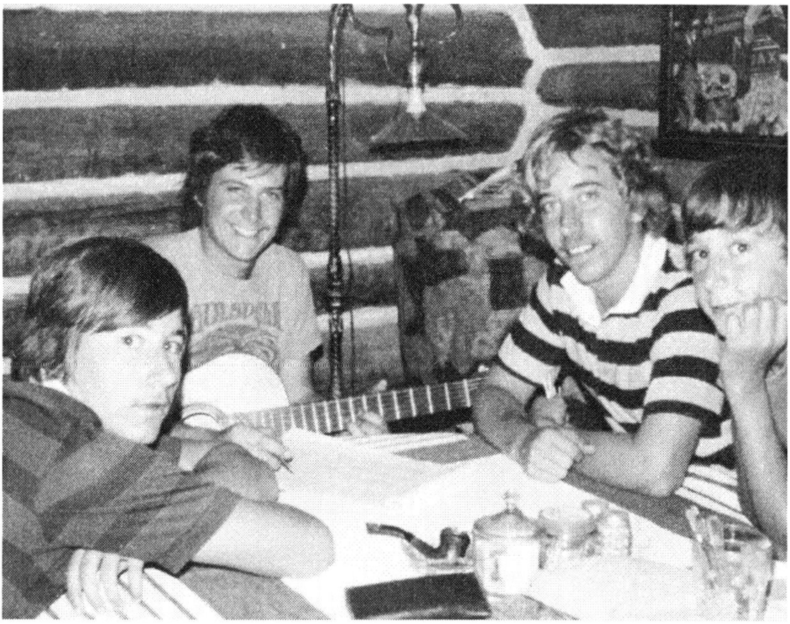

Jim with Bryan and Steve and cousin Tim at Madden's mountain cabin in Creede, Colorado

this day, picturing this episode makes me chuckle—a group of older teenage guys, hoping to enlighten some young teenage kids.

Another time Jim and his friends were invited to a party given by another student. Thinking they'd found the right house, they rang the doorbell and were invited in by the parents. Only after removing their coats did they learn it was the wrong house, the wrong party. The house they were looking for was a few doors away.

The highlight of Jim's high-school years may, perhaps, have been his trip to Germany in 1976. As a Junior, Jim and two very close friends, Bill Hutton and Jim Miettunen, along with others in Mrs. Johnson's German class, participated in the International Student Exchange travel group. They had one great time and a very maturing experience. Jim's German family, the Bergmanns of Pforzheim, became friends to Al and myself, too, as we corresponded with them and visited them several times in Germany.

It was also during Jim's junior year that his cousin, Mary, lived with us while she attended school in the Twin Cities. All of us, including Bryan and Steve, welcomed her presence and humor. Though five years older than Jim, she really bonded with him. After she returned home to Colorado, Jim corresponded with her. When sitting down to write those letters, Jim would really deliberate. After he'd been "writing" a while, he'd say, "Mom, what should I write?" I'd ask, "What have you written so far?" The answer would most often be, "Dear Mary." You need to understand: Jim was a perfectionist; everything he really "got into" had to be done with perfection.

Off to College

When Jim went off to college in the fall of 1977, I felt a real sadness. Even though at the beginning he was just commuting to the University of Minnesota, somehow I knew it was the end of one part of our lives and the beginning of another. We had thought Jim could save money by living at home but he found he was giving up valuable study time in commuting. He even used a cassette recorder to better use that travel time.

It was through Sigma Chi fraternity that Jim found a home on campus. He was introduced to Sigma Chi through a mutual acquaintance of Al's. Jim became a "pledge" and then, an official "Sig." At first he was a "townie," living at the fraternity house only during the school week; later he became a full-time resident. It was here at the fraternity house that Jim got his nicknames, Jimbo Dino and J. D. Jim's years at Sigma Chi were happy ones and he would make many lifelong friends there. These friends were with him both socially and in mutual business ventures. They would later support him when he established his new dental practice. Many of these friends, along with his high school classmates, would become his first patients. (They continue to be for our family, both friends and support in our mutual loss.) Jim's only frustration was that many times when the others in the house were partying, he had to forgo the fun and hide away in his room, studying. Finally, along with two other Sigs, he rented a house off-campus.

Al and I became involved with Sigma Chi, too. The fraternity had a Mothers' Club and I was its president for two years. We had some close years with Jim and Sigma Chi, as we would later when

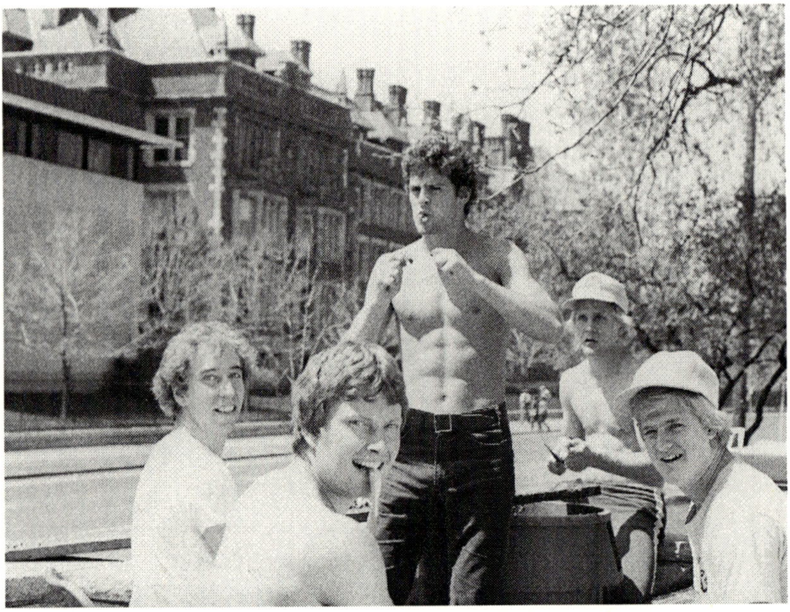

At Sigma Chi Fraternity, cleaning smelt for the annual smelt fry that evening. Filling two garbage cans were: Jim ("Dino"), John Faldin, Mike Yung, Terry Larson, and Layne Chappel. (Photo courtesy of Mike Yung)

Jim's brother, Steve, would join the same fraternity. The big annual events were the Curry Dinners, Sweetheart Teas and balls, which we all attended together.

Jim had continued working at Powers but this meant additional commuting. He was happy when, through one of his Sigma Chi brothers, he was able to get a job with the engineering and consulting firm of Michaud Cooley. He had always liked designing and drawing and though this job involved serving as a courier, he was happy to be in those environs.

When the Sigma Chi pledges kidnapped Jim one Friday from his class at the university, he felt honored. After all, you wouldn't take someone away for a weekend (all the way to North Dakota) if that person wasn't well-liked and fun-loving.

Spring's rite of passage was a trip to Duluth for smelting season. Bryan remembers one of these when Bryan's truck broke down and they had to return home and reload everything into our old, dependable Cadillac. It was a long trek to Congdon Creek and before Bryan had a chance to wet his net, so many fish were netted that he had to return for the car to load the catch of the others. Mike Yung remembers another smelting trip when Jim was caught by the game warden without his fishing license. All of these fishing adventures were followed by an annual smelt fry at the frat house.

When he was still in grade school, Jim, along with his brothers and sisters, had taken lessons in downhill skiing. Now, he had the opportunity to take winter ski trips to Aspen and Vail with his fraternity brothers. There were also fun weekends at the cottages of fraternity parents. Jim's brother, Bryan, remembers going along on one fraternity weekend. When the guys ran out of popcorn, Jim got the idea of trying to re-pop all of the unpopped kernels they had saved! Bryan recounts another outing to a small bowling alley in Tomahawk. When there were no lanes available for them, the management, on Jim's suggestion, allowed them to set up extra pins behind the seating section.

During the years Jim and his brothers were in college, I typed their papers for them. It seemed I was always typing the night before the paper was due. And, I probably issued a warning about last-minute jobs. One time Jim's sister, Jeanne, was either helping me out or bailing Jim out. She ended up at the fraternity house on the day the paper was due, typing the paper as Jim wrote it. The paper, on DNA, was finished and Jim delivered it by sliding the assignment under the professor's door.

Also during his college years, Jim continued singing–something he had always loved to do. A tenor, he had sung in the Hill-Murray High School choir and, later, he would sing in the choir of Edina's St. Patrick's Church. Now, he took voice lessons, and many times he asked me to accompany him on the piano. We did this in the privacy of late evening, so that our mistakes would be less noticed by the family.

In 1981 Jim was chosen to receive the Balfour Award for his

Sigma Chi chapter. This award designates the most outstanding, active graduating senior in the Fraternity. The award recognized Jim for his scholarship, good character, fraternity service, and student (campus) activity. He had also received periodic scholarships from the Fraternity. Al and I have always felt that our sons were in the very best fraternity—one with high ideals.

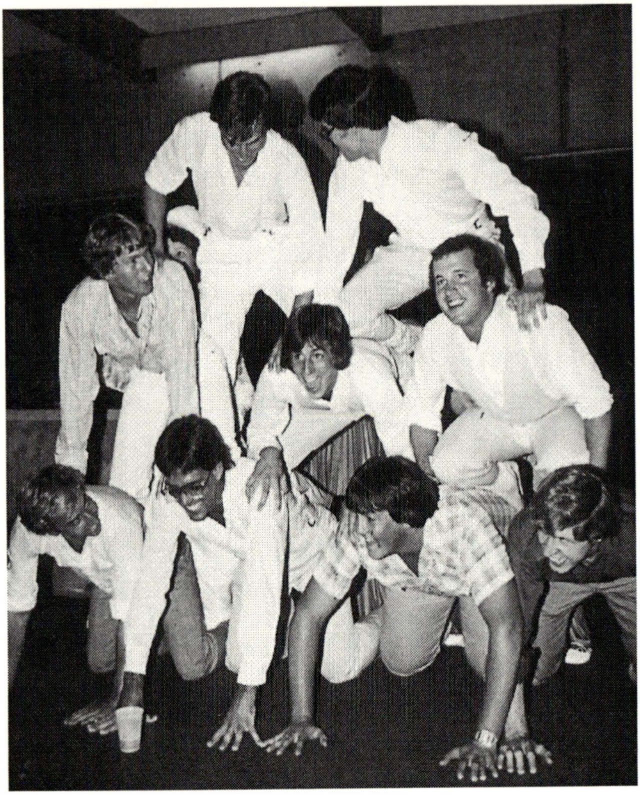

At a friend's wedding in 1981—the human pyramid of bottom row: Jim, friend Dave Paddock, Larry W. and Dick Marty: second row: Jimmy Rieschl, Bill Hutton and Mike Rieschl; top row: Groom Paul Neubauer and Paul Hugo (Photo courtesy of Hill-Murray friends)

Dental School

WHEN JIM BEGAN HIS FOUR YEARS OF DENTAL SCHOOL in 1981, he and another Sigma Chi friend, Randy Larson, bought a house in south Minneapolis. Jim, Randy and the Larson and Deininger families worked together cleaning the bungalow. Jim asked Al for his building expertise and the two families helped in finishing both the second floor and the basement. This gave the investors five bedrooms to rent out—to fellow dental students, fraternity brothers and siblings. At one time, both of Jim's brothers, Bryan and Steve, were renters. The house was just blocks from the Mississippi River and Minnehaha Falls, an area where Jim liked to bike and cross-country ski. Randy's parents lived next door and Mrs. Larson and Jim would go ice-skating together—with Maxine helping Jim perfect his figure-eights and skating backwards.

Ever the optimist, Jim was always cheerful and patient. I must relate two examples of these qualities. During three seasons of the year, he biked to the university from his house. When the Schwinn bike, which he had purchased in Madison with earnings from his paper route, was stolen from the alley garage, he said he was glad that whoever had stolen it had at least left an old bike in its place. On another occasion, he told us of a trip he had made by bike to the post office, late in the afternoon, in the rain, trying to get there before closing time. He didn't realize until he returned home that he had lost his wallet. So he got back on his bike, in the dark, in the rain. He said he was really lucky, because he had found the wallet right under the street light of an intersection.

In the winter months, he drove his used Plymouth, which

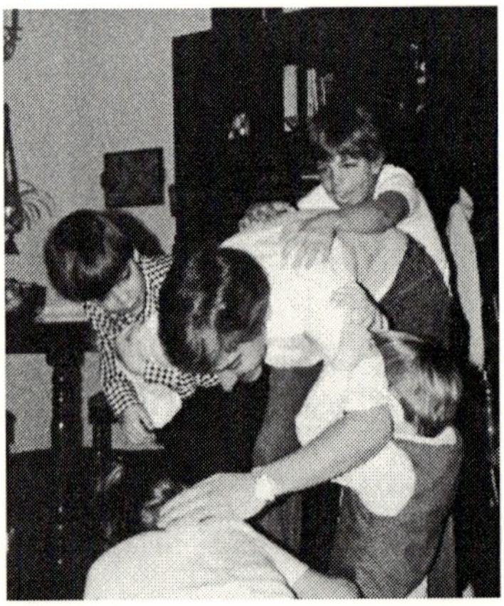

Jim's niece and nephews: Terri, Brian, Brent and Chris Lukens—roughhousing with him in 1983

required real patience. The engine would kill whenever Jim slowed down. It also had no heater. When he and Steve would leave for the university, their warm bodies and recently-shampooed, wet hair fogged the windows. So, in addition to driving without heat, they had to open the windows—all in 20-below-zero weather.

The D.D.S. (Doctor of Dental Surgery) program requires considerable effort and sacrifice to complete and Jim revealed, years later, that he considered getting through dental school one of his greatest successes in life. Jim and his classmates found many ways to break the tediousness of their studies and the daily grind. One day, his fellow classmates gave Jim the nickname Jimbo Billy Bob. Tom DeWitt relates that this led the professor to ask Jim if he was from the South. Jim loved food and he told me about the many times that Linda DeWitt, wife of his dental partner, sent her homemade cookies to school with Tom for them to enjoy.

Diversions were always welcome. On one of his trips home, Jim asked me if I knew of St. Apollonia. I hadn't; so he told me someone in his dental class had learned that St. Apollonia was the patron saint of dentists. This led to their planning a St. Apollonia party one evening. I learned that

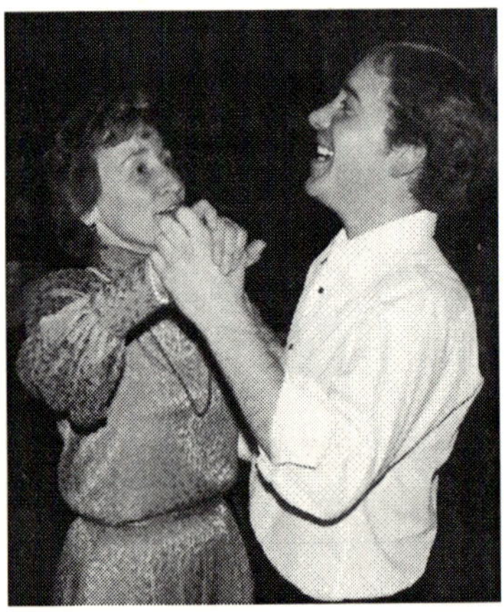

Jim dancing with Mom, 1983

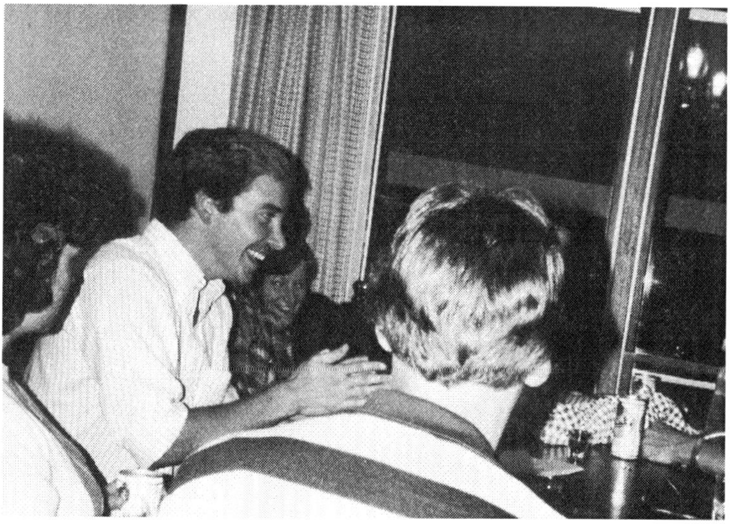

Always the great communicator, Jim enjoyed a captive audience—whether telling a story or performing some kind of trick. 1983, with sister, Jeanne, and brother, Steve

St. Apollonia was a young virgin and martyr whose executioners had broken all her teeth.

During the years he was doing his practicals, Jim was very caring about the patients he had at the university. One year, during a blizzard on the day before Thanksgiving, Jim didn't arrive home when expected. As we waited dinner, the radio warned of the hazardous travel conditions. When he finally arrived home safely, hours later, we learned the reason for his delay. One of his last appointments of the day had been an elderly patient, who left behind his eyeglasses. Concerned that the man would not be able to enjoy his Thanksgiving, Jim had driven in the storm to the man's home and returned his glasses.

Though frugal, Jim's generosity exceeded the contents of his wallet. On a trip to Hennepin County Medical Center, where he was to observe in surgery, he was approached by a street person asking for money. Jim gave him what he had in his pocket—only to find, later, that he had no money left for parking.

In the summer following his third year in dental school, Jim

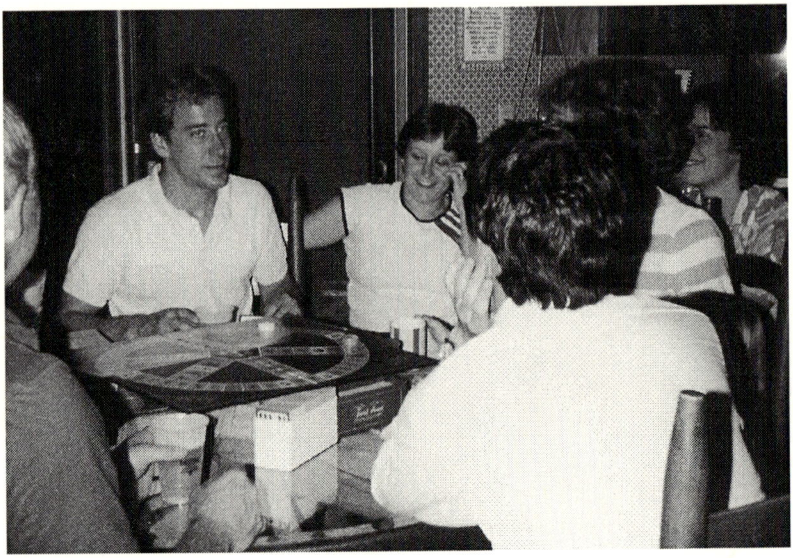

Jim, "staring down" a Trivial Pursuit opponent

was able to get a job with one of the suppliers of dental operatory equipment. At this job, for which he traveled the Twin Cities and southern Minnesota, he had to replace a part on one of the models of dental chairs. One of the dentists whom he called on offered him a partnership. This was one year before his graduation from Dental School! Jim declined; it was his dream to start his own practice.

As the Christmas of 1983 approached, Jim felt the pressures of dental school lessening. With a little more freedom, he declared that this would be the Christmas to "get cultural." He invited Al and me to join him for Tchaikovsky's *Nutcracker* at Northrop Auditorium. On another night we met for a lecture by Prof. Karlis Kaufmanis, "The Star of Bethlehem." During this presentation at the McKnight Omnitheatre, Kaufmanis, a professor emeritus of astronomy at the University of Minnesota, explained his theories on how different constellations and planets may have merged or aligned to form the bright star that, according to the Bible, led wise men to Bethlehem where Jesus was born. Star scenes from

32 B.C. were projected onto the museum's 180-degree concave overhead screen during the lecture. These were both enjoyable evenings and we were most thankful to Jim for his suggestions and for this truly memorable Christmas.

Jim had always been an artist—in grade school, he had done a beautiful painting of autumn trees. In high school, after completing his oil paintings and several pieces of pottery, he began to do some woodcarving. In his fourth year in Dental School, with a little more time to pursue other interests, Jim took on some unique holiday projects. Now, at Halloween in 1984, he carved a pumpkin with a full set of teeth, and braces complete with wires and foils. Then at Christmas, he sculpted nativity figures in the shapes of various teeth. I wish he had taken pictures of them.

I still have the pendant Jim made for me on my birthday. It is my initial "D," which he designed and cast in gold. It was presented in a paper dental cup! I treasure this and wear it always as it is something Jim worked to shape with his own hands.

When Jim was a fourth-year dental student, we had one of our last Merry Christmases, that of 1984. Then, in January, we flew to Colorado for the wedding of Jim's cousin, Guy. Jim sat next to me on the plane and, when I removed my eyeglasses, he noticed the marks left on the bridge of my nose by the glasses. He entreated me, then, to get the contact lenses which I had often spoken about wanting to do. For our anniversary, I received a gift certificate from Al, Jim and Steve for the contacts. It was Jim's idea to write the certificate on "Contact" paper. He seemed always concerned for my well-being and appearance; many times he would buy me clothes (even dresses) as gifts. And, he had good taste in doing so. This would be our last family vacation trip.

A Bittersweet Year

On June 14, 1985, Jim graduated from the University of Minnesota School of Dentistry. We were so very proud of our son as he received his doctorate in the special doctoral robe; he had accomplished so much! Jeanne and Steve were with us for the ceremony, as were Jim's grandparents, who had come from Wausau. Afterwards, we all went to a late dinner at McCormick's, in the Radisson University Hotel; and, then, nearing midnight, we drove to see Minnehaha Falls. This was one of

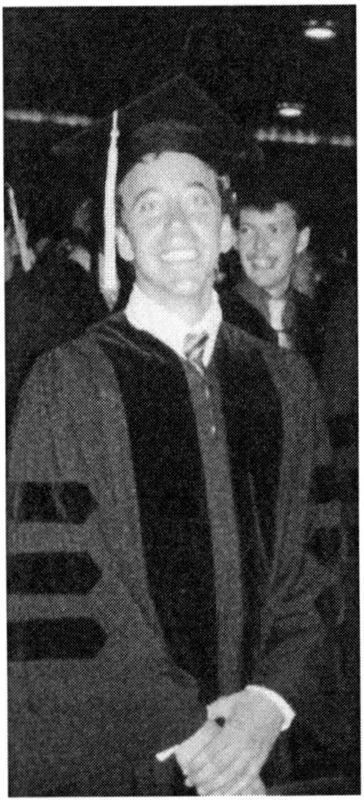

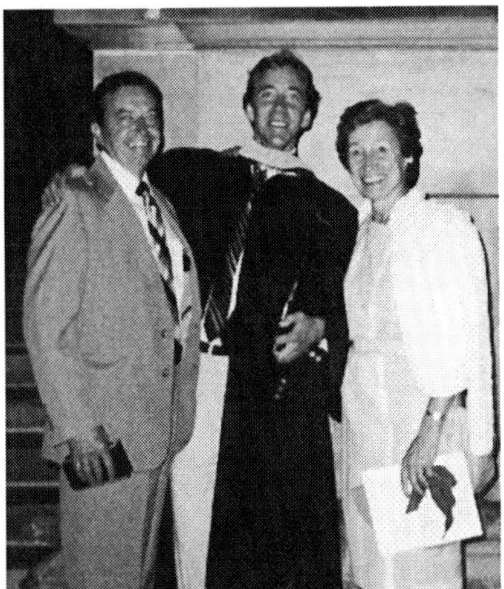

Dr. Jim Deininger, with a very proud Mom and Dad, outside Northrop Auditorium. June 14, 1985

In his doctoral robe, DDS graduation

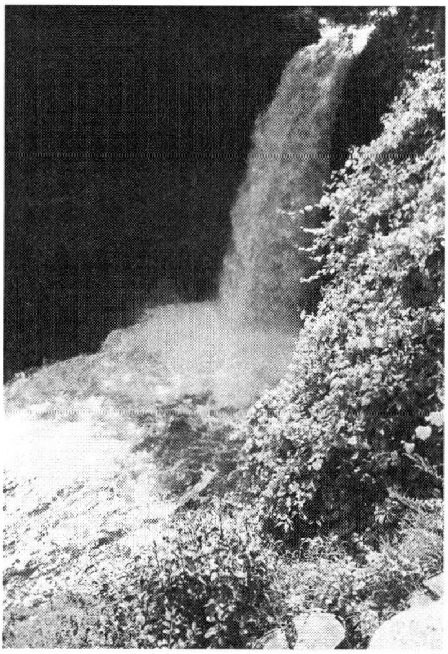

Minnehaha Falls

Jim's favorite places in the Twin Cities and he wanted to share it with us. For his graduation, we gave Jim the bike he had taken to show us a couple of weeks earlier, a French Motobecane Sport, and *The Song of Hiawatha* by Henry Wadsworth Longfellow.

As we approached the celebration of our 35th wedding anniversary and the 60th anniversary of his grandparents, Jim was approaching the state boards for his Degree of Doctor of Dental Surgery. On June 16, after celebrating the anniversaries with us and 100 guests at our cottage in Wisconsin, he and Al returned to Minneapolis for Jim to take his written and practical exams.

The summer was an exciting one. Jim planned to open his own dental practice and enlisted us in his search for just the right location. He had done his demographic homework well and decided to open his practice in Eden Prairie, the fastest-growing suburb of the Twin Cities at that time. I remember noticing several times that summer that Jim seemed under stress. It was very unlike Jim to show stress. One of those periods was preparing for and awaiting the results of his boards. The other was after we returned from a trip to Edmore, North Dakota, where we had gone with Jim to look at some dental fixtures and equipment he hoped to buy. The negotiations fell through (though he would succeed in purchasing the equipment weeks later).

I was concerned at seeing him stressed. But he did all the right things to relax. He exercised on the universal gym he and Steve

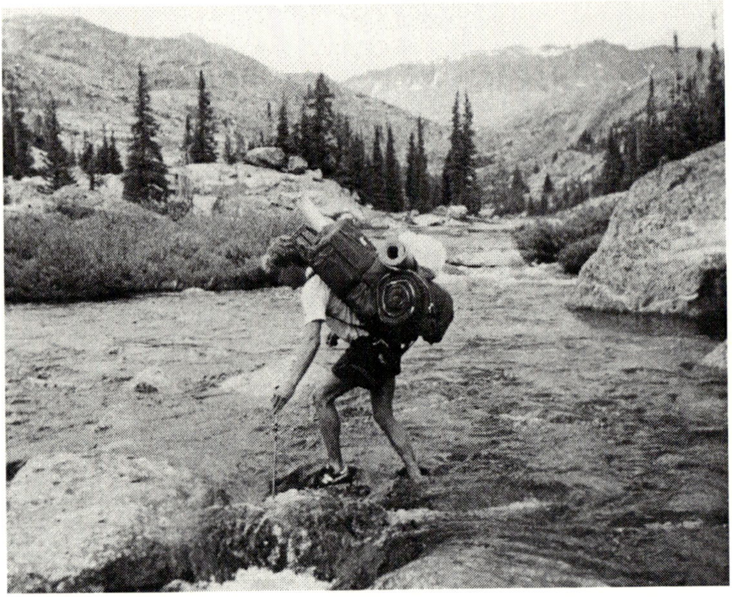

July 1985—Jim, crossing a stream on the backpacking trip to the Big Horn Mountains of Wyoming (Photo courtesy of Eileen Slettebo)

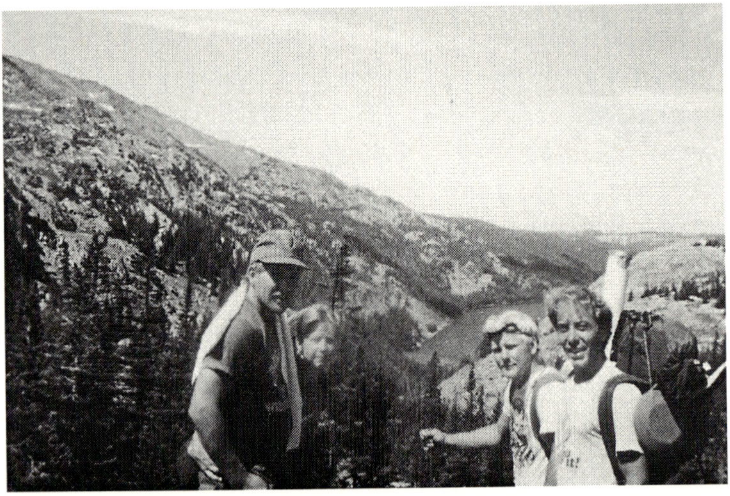

Arriving at "the special place." Brad Larson, Eileen, Terry Larson, and Jim (Photo courtesy of Eileen Slettebo)

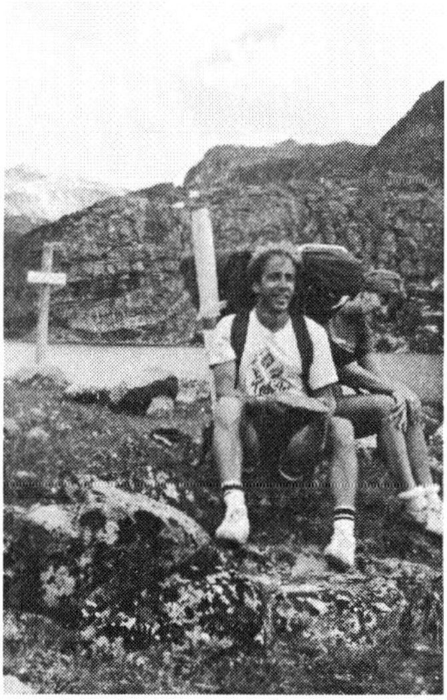

To cross the rushing mountain stream, Jim shared his second pair of shoes with Eileen. (Photo courtesy of Eileen Slettebo)

had built. He took long, 25-mile biking tours. And he had a very good vacation in July, when he accompanied his friends Eileen Slettebo and Brad and Terry Larson on a backpacking, hiking, and fishing adventure to the Big Horn Mountains of Wyoming. Eileen (who died of breast cancer four years after Jim's death) recalled in her travelogue that there would have been "mutiny on the mountain" had it not been for Jim. He supported Brad in his search for the "special place," which led them, after a grueling hike, to "secluded crystal lakes and rare golden trout."

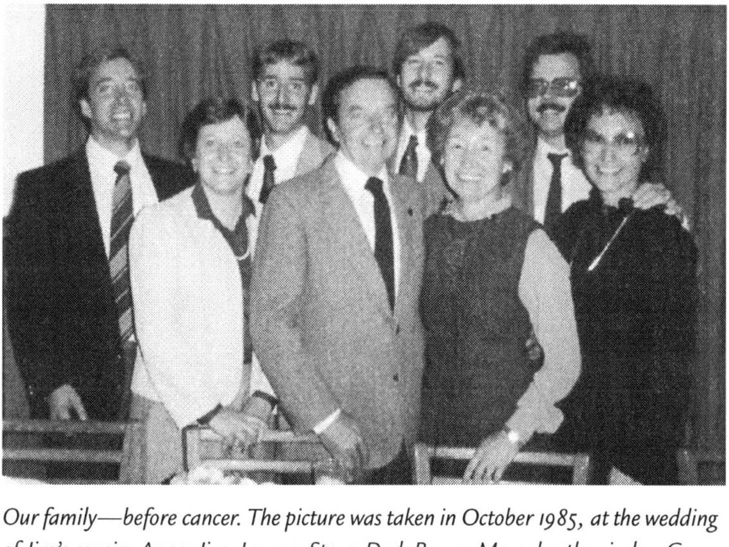

Our family—before cancer. The picture was taken in October 1985, at the wedding of Jim's cousin, Anne: Jim, Jeanne, Steve, Dad, Bryan, Mom, brother-in-law Gary Lukens, Kathy.

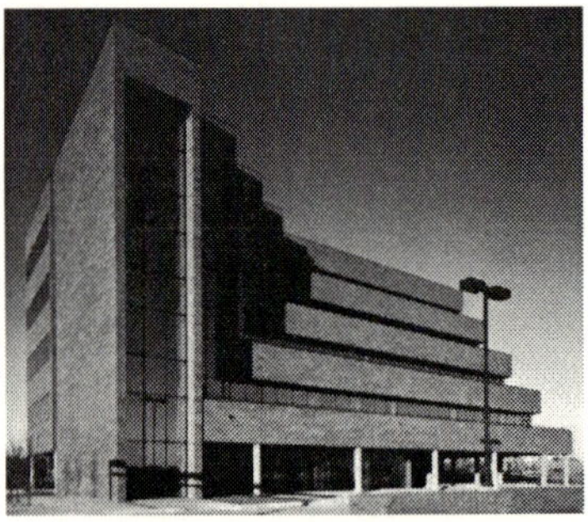

6640 Shady Oak Road, Eden Prairie

In the fall, Jim secured his lease—in a beautiful five-story professional building—and work on his leasehold improvements began. He designed his operatory cabinets and made a floor plan for the operatories and reception and lab rooms. Jim, Al, and I put in some very long days at 6640 Shady Oak Road. Al and a friend made all of the cabinets. And we had fun shopping for the reception room furniture, clocks, and coffee maker. I remember how exciting it was for Jim to order his business cards and brochures. He would have made a good cartographer; he delighted in making maps and charts.

On November 19, Jim hung out his shingle and saw his first patient—a Sigma Chi brother, Greg Notvedt—for an exam and full-mouth x-rays, earning his first $55. Two days later, he held a glorious open house. We were so very proud of Jim!

Just one week later, on Thanksgiving Day, as Jim and Steve were installing a stereo at Jim's office, he felt a lump in his neck. He called home to tell us they would stop at the hospital on their way home to dinner. We hoped the diagnosis would be something like mono. Coincidentally, the day after his open house, Jim had stayed home from the office because he wasn't feeling well. He thought he had the flu, though the vomiting seemed

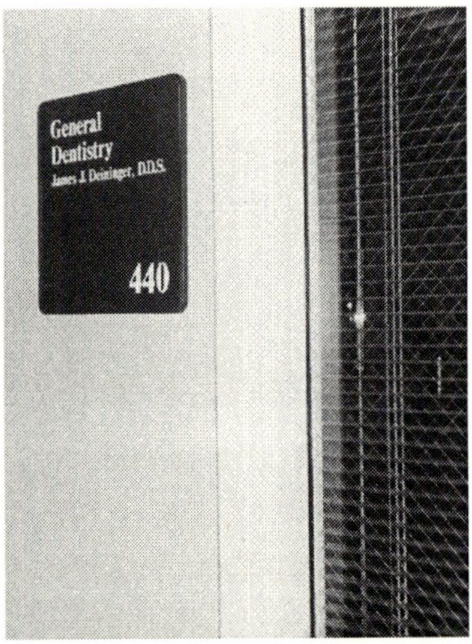

Jim's "shingle"

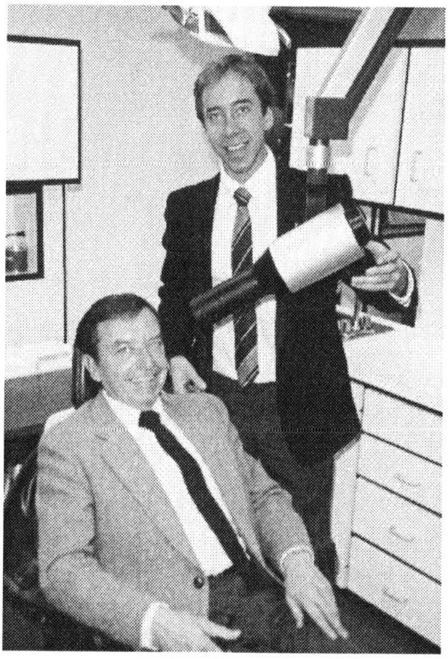

Jim and his Dad at the Open House for Jim's new dental offices, Nov. 21, 1985

unusual as it occurred almost exactly every 45–60 minutes.

After almost a week, when our local hospital and general practitioner provided only a differential diagnosis, Jim went to see an ear-nose-and-throat specialist, Dr. George Adams, at the university. In early December, Jim was admitted to the University of Minnesota Hospital. Both Jim and I were very impressed with Dr. Adams—a skilled surgeon, with an honest and caring manner. He gave Jim several possibilities of what the lump might be, ranging from a benign cyst to much more grave conditions. Surgery and a biopsy revealed the awful news: it was Hodgkin's Disease. "The cancer to have if you're going to have to have cancer," was what many of the medical staff said! It was very difficult and hurt so much to have to reply to our son's question, as he was being returned to his room from surgery, "Yes, Jim, it is cancer." Sensing his anxiety, I asked if he wanted me to stay at the hospital that evening. He said he'd appreciate that, and so I stayed—sleeping in the chair next to our son's bed.

In surgery, during the biopsy, the thoracic duct was accidentally clipped. Consequently, Jim had a drainage tube in his neck. When, twice, the staff overlooked the Doctor's orders and did not follow through with a no-fat diet, the Doctor discharged Jim on the third day, feeling I could be more careful with his diet than they had been at the hospital.

In mid-December, Jim returned to the hospital to determine

the stage of the Hodgkin's. Tests were done, including lymphangiogram and bone marrow biopsy, and the results were good. During this time, it was recommended that Jim have his hepatitis vaccine before the recommended removal of his spleen. Again, orders were not followed and only after my reminder was the vaccine given. I felt a constant need to monitor and be on the alert. On the previous hospitalization, following the diagnosis, a hematologist/oncologist had visited Jim in his room. I was not impressed with her or her manner and I asked Jim if he might want to see another doctor. He seemed satisfied, however, with her assignment to his case. In the following years, during his multiple hospitalizations for surgeries which she had recommended and scheduled, or for infections when they occurred, never once did I see her visit him when he was a patient in the hospital.

The whole family came home for Christmas. The day after Christmas, at 5:00 A.M., I took Jim to the hospital for a laparotomy, spleenectomy and biopsy of the liver. The results were good, though a few affected lymph nodes were found in his chest cavity. Jim was staged at II-A (II because Hodgkin's cells had been found in two areas—the neck and chest; A, because he had experienced none of the classic Hodgkin's symptoms such as nightsweats.) Jim, Al and I were given the news on New Year's Eve and it seemed our prayers were being answered. We celebrated New Year's Eve with Jim in the hospital—"just looking" at the basket of Molson's we had brought him. During this stay, Jim was given Demerol for pain and I never realized, because he seemed so aware of all that happened, that he was actually very "out of it." He said later, that he wasn't even aware of his grandparents coming to visit him in the hospital—though at the time he had carried on a normal conversation with them.

Another oversight occurred at this time. I had read, and we had been told, that before Jim's recommended radiation, he visit a cryogenic lab—for sperm to be taken and frozen. However, no orders were written and only when I reminded the doctor and staff of this, did they follow through.

Between the time of Jim's hospitalizations for surgery and the beginning of his radiation, he would encounter yet another stressful battle. In the fall of 1984, The Minnesota Dental Association (MDA) had given a recognition-type dinner to the fourth-year students of the Dental School. At that time, he received a free membership in the MDA. When Jim had called the MDA to sign up for the group insurance plan, he was given the Blue Cross/Blue Shield brochure but told that he had missed the 40-day-limitation deadline for coverage—a circumstance created only by the fact that he'd had the complimentary membership. Jim had not been aware of this time limitation because during the time he had the complimentary MDA membership, he never received the insurance brochure giving the sign-up deadline. Consequently, he had to sign up for insurance coverage through the state—until his attorney was able to win for him an individual Blue Cross/Blue Shield plan.

From January through April of 1986, Jim underwent his prescribed radiation treatment—both upper and lower mantle, to the neck and chest areas. From all I had read at the University Medical Library, this was the recommended treatment of the time. In retrospect, I believe that an adjuvant treatment of chemotherapy, at that time, might perhaps have been a saving treatment—because of the affected nodes found in the chest cavity.

Halfway through the radiation treatment, Jim took a week off and flew to Puerto Vallarta, Mexico. He had received this all-expense-paid trip for having

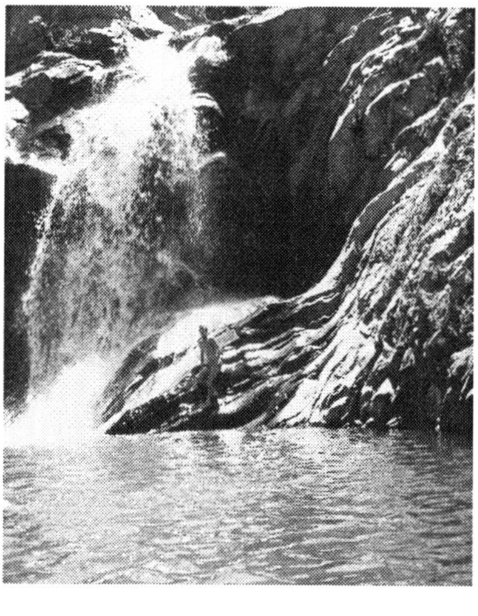

March 1986. Jim's trip to Puerto Vallarta, Mexico—in the middle of his four-month radiation treatment

attended a sales pitch at Breezy Point Resort with us the previous summer. The trip was good for him. He went hang-gliding and had a much-needed and deserved rest. When we picked him up at the airport, his color was good.

During this period of radiation, Jim experienced fatigue and some loss of hair at the neckline. One day as I was assisting chair-side, I noticed for the first time the hairs on his lab coat collar, and I felt a pang of pain, as Jim had always had a beautiful head of hair. I never suspected the poking, prodding and cutting that would be part of his future. After his early-morning treatment, Jim often went home to rest and came into the office to work half days. In November he had answered an ad to housesit for a couple in Edina who wintered in Florida. Their home was only about two miles from the office so the location was ideal. Steve stayed there with Jim for the first two weeks after his discharge from the hospital.

We began, then, to build the new practice. Jim had a good business head and was a skilled and compassionate dentist. I know from first-hand experience because I was both his office manager and his dental assistant—as well as a patient, of course! My offer to volunteer in his office had led to my role as receptionist/office manager. After his diagnosis, Jim trained me as his dental assistant, also. "It'll be good for your resume," he jokingly said. One of the first things he did was design his own crown remover, which Steve built for him. In his years of practice, this was an often-used instrument.

Jim had been given a prognosis of a 90-95 percent cure-rate. He was feeling very positive and had "the world on a string." When he wasn't with appointments, we did all forms of marketing and we practiced relaxation and mental imagery in the empty chair. Later, I would find one of Jim's journal entries from 1986, with reference to *The Chronicles of Narnia*: "Aslan is within me. When comparing myself with the ideal, I am that ideal." He was striving to win the battle. He would have three successful, happy years.

The Dentist and His Assistant

In the four years he had in his dental practice, Jim and I worked daily side-by-side. We had a good rapport and he usually called me "Dona." But when patients did learn of our mother-son relationship, they often commented, "No wonder you work so well together!" I don't know of any son and mother who spent as much time together as we did, philosophizing and working together those four years. I am so thankful for that. In our unusually strong relationship, I was mother, fellow worker, and caregiver. The first two roles gave me much joy; the latter gave me hope.

Funny as it may sound, Jim held staff meetings for the two of us. Some who knew of this found it amusing and a bit out of the ordinary. But know that Jim was not ordinary. He knew that these meetings would give us the opportunity and time to discuss mental notes and to openly state our feelings in a business-like setting. When the first Secretaries' Day rolled around in April, I was pleasantly surprised to receive flowers and be taken out to lunch. On National Boss Day in October, I reciprocated.

New patients, of course, had to fill out a chart—filling in the usual informational I.D., along with other specific dental history questions. When one of Jim's colleagues, Dr. Tom DeWitt, came in to do Jim's own dental exam, Jim, too, filled out a new chart. Afterward, when I was charting the exam, I noticed that in answer to "Reason for visit," Jim had filled in, "I work here."

We also spent many hours marketing his practice. In four years he would build his practice to 500 patients. Jim always felt it would be better to spend unfilled chair time for marketing, rather than having another part-time job at another practice or at the Dental School. In just three years he was able to pay off his business loan of $46,000 and realize a net profit of $35,000.

His best marketing tool, next to his ability as a dentist, was his closeness to every one of his patients. Beginning with his very first patient, he appreciated each one, spent time with each person without being rushed, and knew everyone by name. And Jim had such very nice patients. We truly enjoyed their company. Soon, referrals became the main builder of our patient base.

Jim also began a breakfast-study club for fellow dentists, which met one morning a month in our building. It began at 7:30 A.M. with a continental breakfast, followed by a speaker. The lectures gave attendees continuing-education credits. Maclin Dental Laboratory helped us with mailings and meeting set-ups. Jim was always conscious of his dental posture and one of the speakers was a patient of ours who was a physical therapist. He presented a program on the posture of dentists to prevent occupational back problems. In addition, Jim belonged to another monthly breakfast club organized by one of his Sigma Chi brothers. They met in Minneapolis and surrounding suburbs for the purpose of networking.

One of Jim's marketing strategies was a direct mailing to new residents in the zip code areas near his office. We did these about twice a year. The package included a welcoming letter overprinted on letterhead stationery, hand-typed salutations and envelopes, and an informational brochure and business card. It was all done with class. "No coupon offers," Jim said. That patient might easily transfer to the next coupon offer received. Other examples of his personal touch were birthday greetings to patients, a flower of the day for those who had had a difficult procedure performed, or a prized rose he may have brought from his garden.

Though I commuted close to 70 miles a day, I enjoyed every minute of those years. I took great satisfaction in seeing our son working at his profession with his beautifully skilled, deft hands, and being a part of his work in the pleasant surroundings which he'd created. We had a close atmosphere with our landlord, The James Company, and fellow tenants. On the evenings we had appointments, after the patients and other tenants had left, Jim would crank up the stereo to unwind as we did the sterilization and operatory cleanup. Even the drive through city traffic was, for me, both invigorating and contemplative—a time to think, as I made the transition from office to home. We always left the office together. I can still see Jim exiting the Crosstown at Tracy Avenue, only about two miles from the office. Sitting erect in the Olds Cutlass, and with a smug grin on his face, he would give me a wave—as I continued my longer journey home. That mental image remains after these ten years and brings a smile each time I visualize it.

Our landlord, The James Company, was great to us, through both happy days and trying times. Jim's initial introduction was to Charles James, and he worked closely with him in securing his lease. In August of 1986, the Jameses took Jim and some other tenants and business acquaintances on a fun fishing trip to Canada.

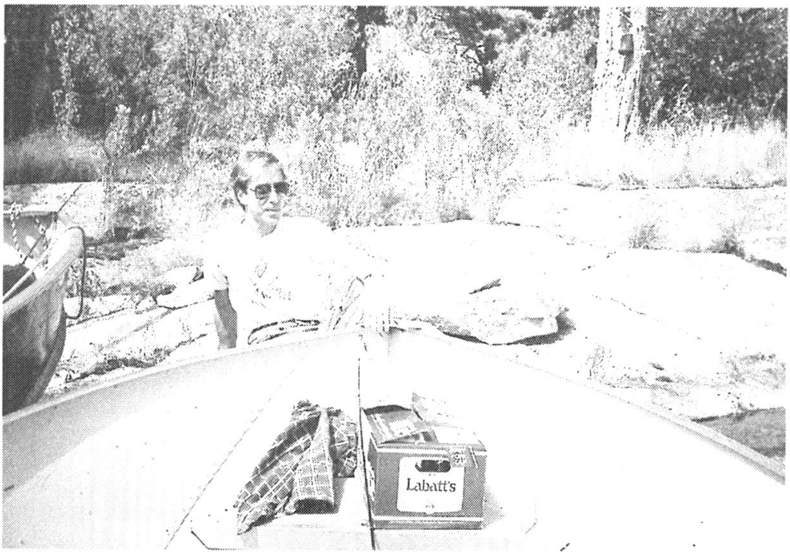

Taken on his fishing trip to Canada with The James Company, August 1986 (Photo courtesy of Bob James)

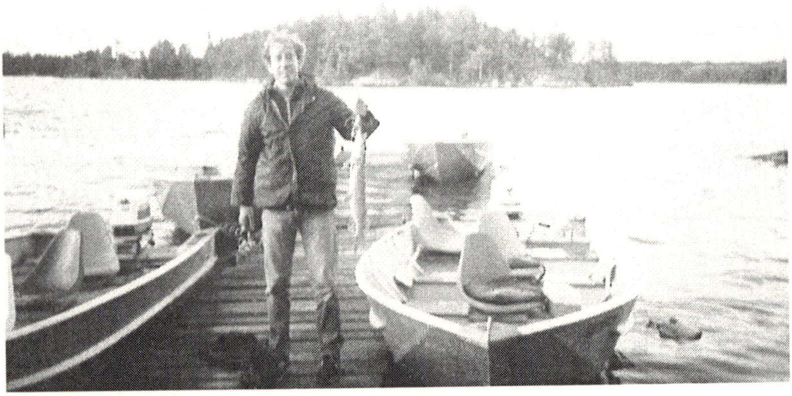

A catch of the day (Photo courtesy of Bob James)

He had a great time; and Bob James never ceased teasing Jim about his tremendous appetite. This would be Jim's vacation for the year; being frugal and of limited financial resources, he made these and other free respites his vacations. Both Jim and I enjoyed the day-to-day business and personal relationship we had with Charlie and the rest of the James family—as well as with Elaine, their receptionist and personal secretary. During Jim's bone-marrow transplant and months of hospitalization in Madison, the "James Gang" lightened the load considerably when Doug James told us we would be given six months of rent-free tenancy.

In the spring of 1986, Jim and Randy Larson had decided to sell their 45th Avenue-bungalow in Minneapolis. Jim asked Al and me to help him search for a house, and throughout the weekends of autumn we did this. Jim knew he couldn't manage another loan at the time and so he wanted a house with a contract-deed advantage. He also wanted it located within a four-mile radius of his practice. We had fun together finding it—a walkout rambler on Wilryan Avenue in Edina. In the meantime, Jim and Steve had lived at home with us for most of the time between April and December. One of the things I miss most is our camaraderie at the dinner table. We often ended up with volumes of the encyclopedia on the table, following some interesting discussion that needed research. In addition to this intellectual stimulation, we would find ourselves in tears of laughter, with Jim and Steve acting as catalysts to each other's humor. Oh, the times were good.

As with the first house, Jim's new abode would have to pay its own way. So he set about designing the lower, walkout level for his own residence. He planned the floor space as he wanted it—two bedrooms, bath, a living room, kitchenette and laundry-storage room. Al pitched in again and Jim's grandfather, who always enjoyed helping his children and grandchildren with their carpentry and remodeling, came from Wausau. Before construction began, however, Jim and Steve had their usual fun by acting as demolition crew. Before long, Jim's tenants were helping provide the monies for his mortgage and taxes.

The latter part of 1986 and all of 1987 were, for Jim, a return to normalcy. His energy was back and the practice was running very smoothly. He began dating and was able to enjoy a full social life with his friends. And our family was blessed with normal holidays at Thanksgiving and Christmas. After Christmas, Jim took some time off and he and Steve flew out to Tahoe for a skiing vacation

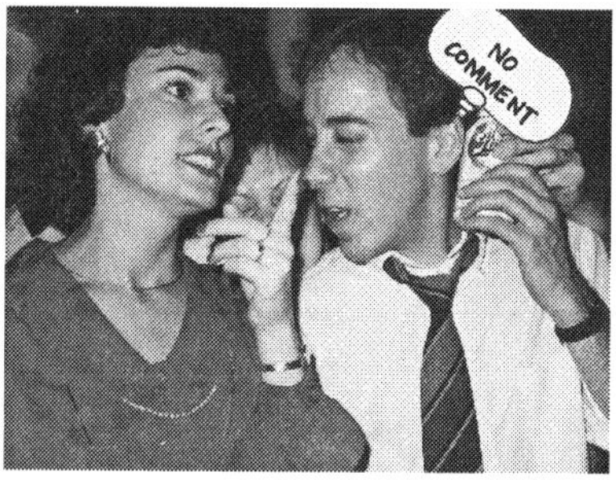

At the wedding of friend Dick Marty: April Paddock and Jim, November 1986 (Photo courtesy of Hill-Murray friends)

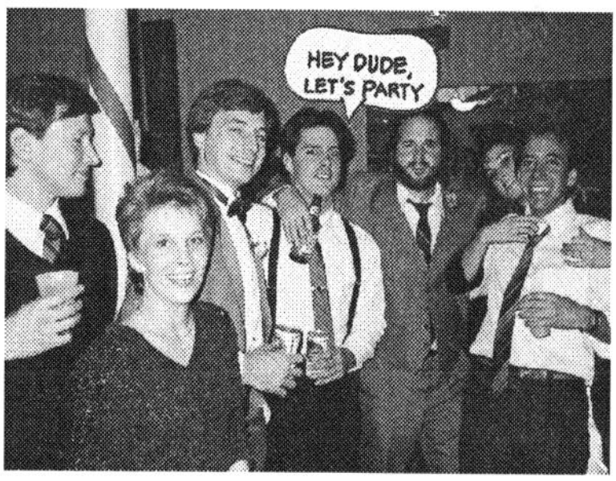

At Marty wedding: Pete Day, Mary Marty, Jim Miettunen, Mark Hales, Mike Rieschl, Kris Kieland, and Jim (Photo courtesy of Hill-Murray friends)

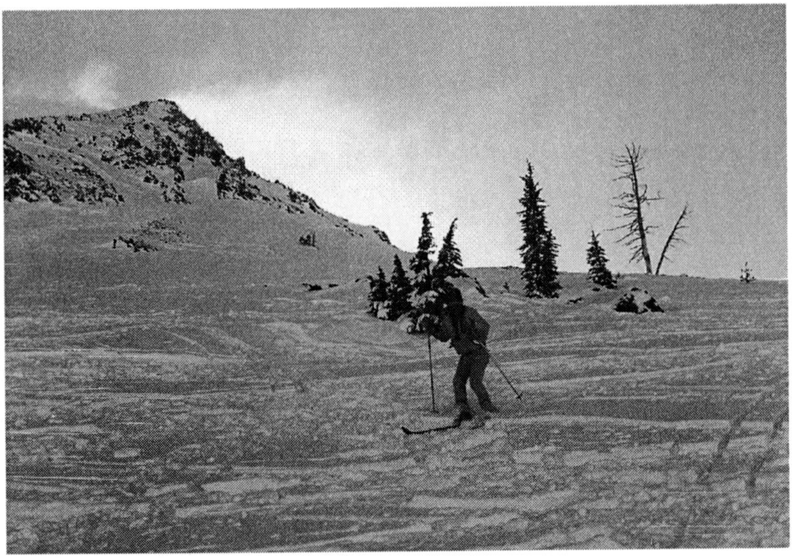

Jim, on a ski trip with brother, Steve, to the resorts of Tahoe. December 1987

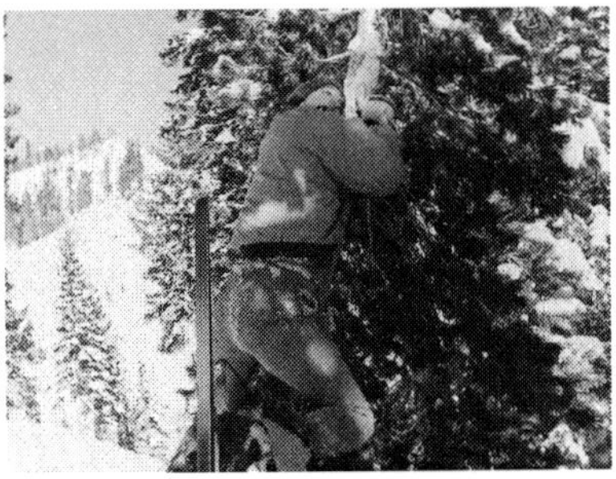

Jim, "hamming it up"—on the Tahoe Trip

with a fraternity friend, Mike Yung. Though Jim had experienced a cough during this holiday time, his doctor was not concerned.

These enterprising brothers had another experience in the previous summer of 1987 when the Twin Cities was experiencing a drought. One evening when Jim and Steve had gone out to buy a lawnmower, the drought was reversed. It began to rain as they left the store and by the time they got to France Avenue, a flash flood had begun. Visibility was not good and when they hit the second wall of water, the car died. When they opened the doors, they soon realized that was not to be the way out. They were able to close the doors and then used the windows to make their exit. After pushing Steve's car into Byerly's lot, they went into the store to buy plastic bags which they used both as rainwear and waders, secured around their waist with duct tape. They walked the approximate two-mile distance to Jim's house, through water knee-to-waist high. The car was totaled. The experience made for a good story that received much mileage.

Jim was especially proud, during this time, to write a letter of recommendation on behalf of Steve, who was applying to the University of Minnesota's Institute of Technology. When Steve won admission, Jim was delighted because he knew a mechanical engineering degree would give Steve the career he was meant to pursue.

In 1988 Jim decided to try an insurance capitation plan. It was very frustrating for both of us. The stress, and working some extra hours at another practice on a temporary basis, though in happy social surroundings, kept Jim running. Because there were so many named Jim at the practice, he again became "Jimbo Billy Bob." Most of his nicknames seemed to include "Jimbo."

One very vivid memory of this July lingers. Ironically, as Al and I rode back to the Twin Cities after a boat trip down the St. Croix and Mississippi Rivers with Joan and Ron Janssen, I was suddenly overwhelmed with a feeling of my life being really blessed. I remember recounting to Al all the things I was thankful for: our family and wide circle of friends, the varied experiences and trips we had managed, and the fact that Jim was approaching three years after his diagnosis. The only shadow was a cough I had heard when I spoke to Jim on the phone one day. I asked him to call his doctor about this.

In October Jim had another CAT scan. He was told that the scan was "o.k." and we were thankful once again. Then, a week later, on October 16, his oncologist called to say they had forgotten to read part of the scan and they had now found something questionable in an area of his chest. She asked him to check into the hospital immediately for surgery the following morning. As we waited in the admissions office, Jim expressed his fear.

From this day forward, for nearly two years, we went from one crisis to another. In late October, Jim had two surgeries: first, a median sternotomy, and then, a mediastinostomy. These were severe and drastic explorative surgeries that involved cutting through Jim's sternum, as is done for open-heart surgery. Jim had always kept himself in excellent physical condition. It was so very difficult for me as a mother to see our son's body cut open again and again. As before, I was with Jim daily at the hospital. At home I was able to retrieve phone messages and reschedule appointments.

I remember one particular afternoon when Jim really poured his heart out—sharing with me his innermost thoughts, intimate feelings and regrets, and necessary plans. This was so difficult for him to be going through, so heart-wrenching for a mother to hear. The surgeons visited during their rounds, the oncologist did not. I remember our long walks through the halls and tunnels of the University Hospital and adjacent buildings. Jim was most

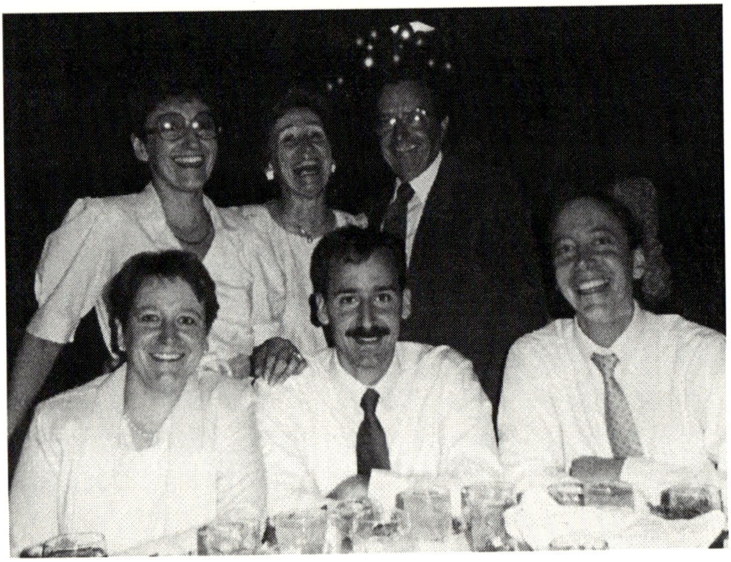

At a Janssen wedding in 1989: Kathy, Dona and Al; Jeanne, Steve, and Jim. Though beginning to lose hair as a result of the chemo, Jim was enjoying this "night out" with his family.

familiar with the university and environs and he put many miles on the wheels of his IV poles. When weather allowed, we walked outside and it bothered him when I had to help move the IV pole over the uneven surfaces of the courtyard. He did not relish losing his independence. Days of waiting became weeks before Jim was told they had found some necrotic cells. And then, a ten-month regimen of chemotherapy was advised.

Jim was, understandably, reticent about the chemotherapy, especially after being told that it could cause other cancers to surface. In December, however, he decided to proceed with the recommended 10-month regimen. The drugs were in alternating cycles of MOPP (a combination of mechlorethamine, vincristin, procarbazine and prednisone) and ABVD (a combination of doxorubicin, bleomycin, vinblastine, and dacarbazine.) These treatments were almost weekly, depending on what his blood count revealed. Given by intravenous drip, they took a couple of hours.

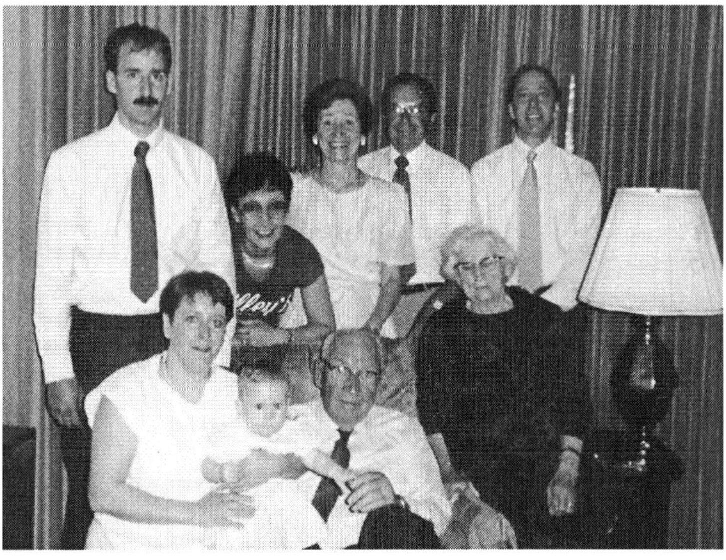

At the Lukens home in Stoughton, Wisconsin: Jim's sister, Jeanne, and her daughter, Amanda; Jim's grandparents, August and Agnes Kraimer. Back row: Jim's brother, Steve; sister, Kathy; Mom, Dad and Jim

Jim insisted on driving himself for his first treatments. He returned home and, after his first few treatments, even pushed himself to go ice-skating—though he said the kids in the warming house looked at him questioningly when, after putting on his skates, he returned five minutes later to take them off again.

The potency of the drugs seemed to build, however. Once in January, the nurses had to call a taxi for Jim's return trip home. He conceded that he could no longer drive himself home from these treatments. He would drive to the hospital, and either Steve or Al would drop me off so that I would be there to drive Jim home in his car. As Jim and I visited during the two-to-three-hour wait for his blood-count results and the ordering of the drugs, we would take walks along the Mississippi River. Then after the couple of hours it took for his chemo "drip," I would claim the car at the ramp, pick him up, and drive him home to his house. It was really heart-wrenching to see our son get so violently sick each week as we made the drive back to his home. Usually so erect, so proud, Jim was now bent over in pain and there was nothing I could do, save praying for his complete recovery. Now, I could only see him to his room as he rested and fought the nausea. Then I went on to the office to work and await Al or Steve to pick me up for our drive home.

Jim's chemo treatments were mid-week and so we would schedule the majority of his patients for early in the week, setting aside the latter part of the week for recovery. In our absence, the answering machine referred emergency patients to one of Jim's colleagues, Dr. Tom Garvin. On occasion, we had to engage another dentist to come in and help us out. At the time, my schedule seemed normal; looking back, I think I must have been running on nervous energy. Love really does transmit strength.

During Jim's course of chemotherapy, my father was hospitalized several times for surgery. Many times, after taking Jim home from his chemo and finishing at the office, I drove the 190-mile drive to Wausau to visit my dad and stay with my mother for a night or two. It was difficult for me to leave Jim but he insisted that I should visit his grandparents. I remember on one trip arriving at the hospital late in the evening. As the main doors had closed around 10 P.M., I had to enter through the emergency room. As I did, I saw a body being wheeled out on a gurney. It was a long, running pace for me before arriving at my father's room. He was sleeping and after I sat several minutes beside his bed, Dad woke and I was greeted with his usual, "Oh, Dona Mae, you're here."

Between surgery and chemo, Jim had decided to sell his practice. Believing he would not be able to continue working throughout the chemo, he inventoried all the equipment and supplies. Afterward, he sat in the operatory chair, just staring out the window. I wondered if he was thinking of all he had put into this practice. After getting an appraisal, he did list it. But, after receiving just one offer, and this for half the valuation—from a peer who was aware of the circumstances—he decided to continue

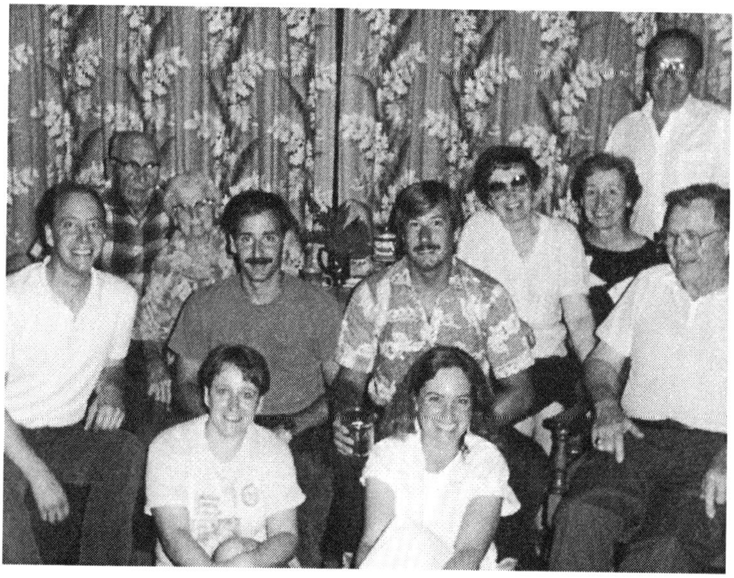

Still on chemo, and facing lung surgery in a few days: Jim and his grandparents; brothers Steve and Bryan; aunt, Rita Madden; Dona and Al; and uncle, Jim Madden. Front row: sister Jeanne; cousin, Mary Madden

working. Two to three days of each week were lost to treatment, but Jim managed to maintain his practice during the balance of the week.

In July Jim had another setback. His oncologist reported another "questionable" spot in the lung area after a nodule was noted on a chest CT scan. About this time, I again asked Jim if he wanted to get another opinion. We knew of an acquaintance of friends in Madison, Wisconsin, who had Hodgkin's Disease and who was very pleased with his oncologist there. Jim thought about it but decided, instead, to talk to another doctor at the University of Minnesota, then continued with his oncologist.

This time she scheduled a thoracotomy of the left lung. I shall never forget how our son looked as he returned from surgery, hooked up to life-support systems and monitors. Jim's body had now been cut open front, side and back–through the neck, the abdomen, the breastbone, and now the thorax and lung. After this surgery, Jim was in the Intensive Care Unit. Because I could

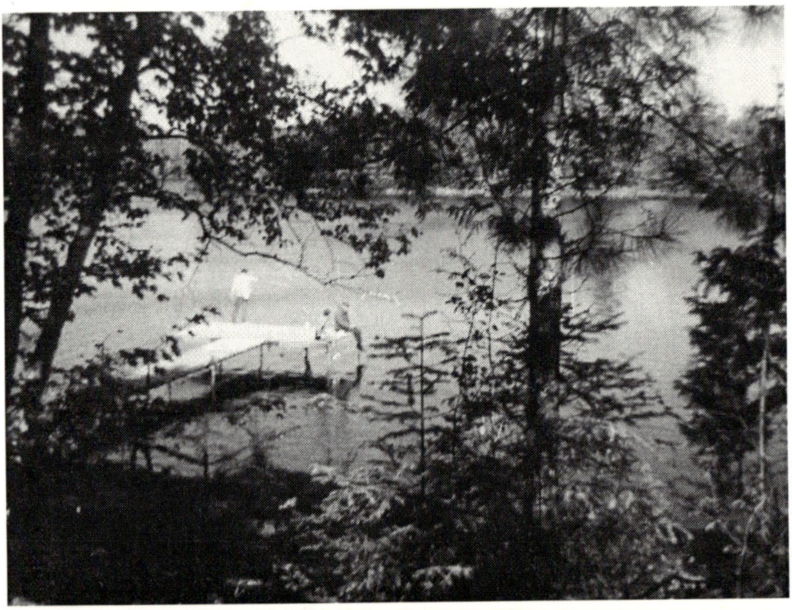

Jim, sitting on the dock, visiting with his grandfather—as Steve fished

not, of course, stay overnight in the ICU room, Al talked me into coming home. But I could not finish the twenty-mile trip; it just seemed too far from our son. So I turned around and returned to the hospital. When I looked in on Jim, he was sleeping. I told the nurse I would be staying, and spent the night sitting in the ICU lounge. I just felt so much better being close to Jim at this critical time.

Several days later as Jim was recovering from the surgery, he sensed something else was wrong. Tests were done and they revealed a pulmonary embolism in his leg. After the tests it was imperative that Jim lie very still and force fluids throughout the evening. I spent the night in his hospital room so that I could wake him regularly to drink water and juices. This development also necessitated therapeutic anticoagulation. The thoracotomy proved the area to be negative for infection or tumor, I was told. In August, Jim resumed practicing; chemo began again in September.

In late September of 1989, a few days following one of his last

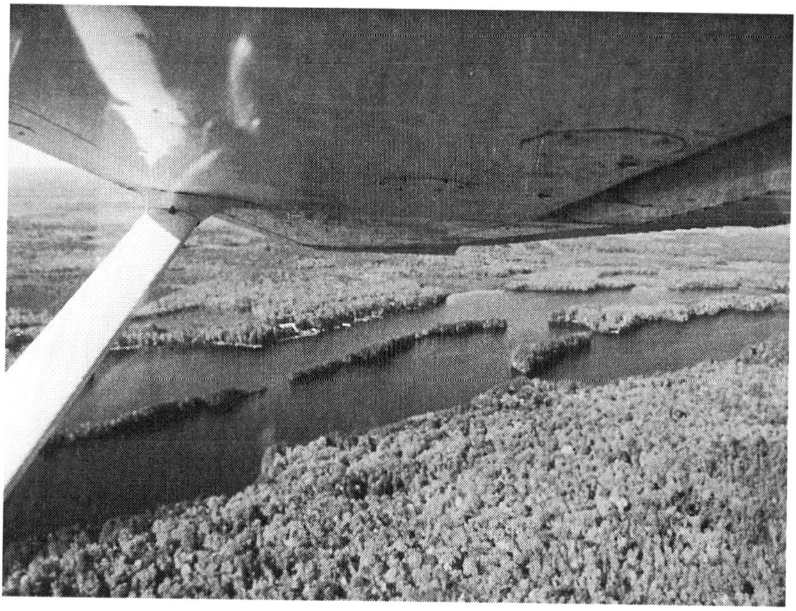

One of the pictures Jim took of Lake Somo on his fly-over in September of 1989

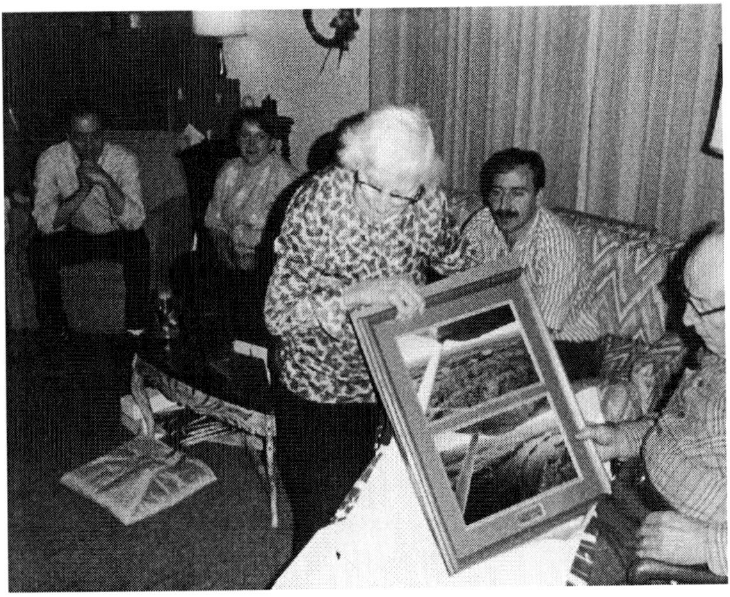

Presenting his grandparents with the framed pictures he'd taken of their lakefront, Jim was most proud. Christmas 1989. Three days later, we would leave for the University of Wisconsin, Madison, for the harvesting of Jim's bone marrow.

chemotherapy treatments, Jim flew to Tomahawk, Wisconsin with one of his renters, who wanted to get some air hours in before getting his pilot's license. They were going to fly over our family cottage, Jim would take some pictures, then they would return home for some afternoon appointments Jim had scheduled at the office. But the combination of his recent treatment, some air turbulence, and the maneuvering of the camera made him so nauseous that they had to put down at an airport in Phillips, Wisconsin.

Jim called the office so that I could reschedule the patients and I arranged for an uncle of mine, who lived near Phillips, to pick Jim up at the airport. When Uncle Bernard walked into the terminal, he took one look at Jim, whom he hadn't seen since he was a toddler, and said, "You must be Jim. You look like your dad." In his usual good humor, Jim replied, "You must be Uncle

Bernard. You look like my grandpa." My parents drove to pick up Jim from my uncle's home and we left to meet the three of them at the cottage.

The photographs Jim took on that trip turned out spectacularly. For Christmas, Jim gave to his grandparents a matted and framed picture of two of his shots. He had always been a thoughtful giver. If he could think of the perfect gift, and he usually did, the cost was never too great.

In October of that year, when his renters—two chiropractic students and a teacher—went their separate ways, Jim decided it was time to treat himself, move upstairs, and rent the walkout level. He would have only two months' residency there to enjoy. For later that month, his oncologist became wary of an elevated monocyte count.

On Nov. 14 another CAT was done. On November 22, the day before Thanksgiving, during what Jim thought was a routine office visit, he learned the seriousness of his condition. There was an increase in size of the anterior mediastinal mass and the development of a pleural-based mass. Jim's doctor told him he might die. I was furious that our son had to hear this news, and that he had to hear it alone. Never did his oncologist indicate I should come with Jim to this visit—though she called later to say she thought I'd be there. Jim had always gone to his regular routine visits alone. How were we to know this one would be different? Everything that was done at the University of Minnesota Hospital Clinic, by staff doctors, was done without an ounce of compassion. We received that compassion only from the surgeons and nurses.

Jim returned to the office just in time for his waiting appointments. It wasn't until after he had seen two patients that he could share with me what he had been told. I shall never forget my son's face at that moment, nor shall I ever forget his words: "Mom, I may die!" These remain etched in my heart for the rest of my days. All I could do was hold him and say, "No, Jim; we shall do what next must be done." And so we talked of the now-planned bone marrow transplant (BMT). As we walked to our cars in the parking level that evening, Jim said to me, "Mom, this body seems so okay. I look and feel fine, but I'm getting so disgusted with all that's going on inside it. And I don't seem to be able to do anything about it." The Hodgkin's disease and its treatments would ravage his body, without curing.

That awful day, I cried all through the 33-mile drive home. I was still crying when I walked into the house. Alarmed, Al asked if I had had an accident. I told him Jim's terrible news. Quietly he said, "Now I wish you had had an accident." One week later, I did.

As I stopped for a traffic light outside White Bear Lake, an inattentive driver, who hadn't noticed the traffic had stopped, "plowed" into me. Because I had left a car's length between me and the truck ahead, I did not hit that truck. Though our car was nearly totaled, I suffered no injuries. Luckily, minutes after the police arrived, Steve happened to be coming home on that same route, and I had some caring assistance.

Prayers and Hope

DURING THIS TIME, JIM AND I WENT TO DAILY MASS. WE would meet at one parish or another, at one time of the day or another, depending on our scheduled appointments. We remained optimistic always, believing each setback would be the last battle to overcome.

As I had twice in the past—before he began chemotherapy, and again at the time of his thoracotomy—I again entreated Jim to see another doctor or to go to the Mayo Clinic or the University of Wisconsin Comprehensive Cancer Center. With the latest development, he considered my plea.

We again called our friends in Madison, whose friend had been diagnosed with a more advanced stage of Hodgkin's. His young and very caring oncologist at the University of Wisconsin Hospital was Dr. Walter Longo. Jim made an appointment with Dr. Longo and, on the weekend after Thanksgiving, Al and I, Jim and Steve drove to Stoughton, Wisconsin. We stayed with Jim's sister, Kathy, and her husband, Gary Lukens and their family. This would be our "home-away-from-home" for the next seven months. Jim brought a small portion of his myriad of medical records from the University of Minnesota. On Sunday Al and Steve returned to Minnesota and Jim and I stayed over for Jim's Monday appointment. Dr. Longo concurred that the autologous bone marrow transplant was the only potential curative form of treatment. Chemotherapy alone, or in combination with radiotherapy, would have no potential for cure, only for short remissions. We drove home with so much hope. Though we were driving through a snowstorm, we were on a real "high" the whole way.

Back in Minnesota, I went with Jim to a previously-scheduled appointment at the University Hospital Clinic. We met with the oncologist and the doctor who would do the bone marrow transplant. He kept interrupting his speaking to throw his head back, in an effort to remove his long hair from his forehead. As we were speaking with the oncologist, the BMT doctor went out into the hall to speak with another doctor. Without closing the door after him, he engaged in a conversation with this doctor, and spoke of another patient who, after having undergone a life-threatening BMT, had "relapsed again." Ethics and compassion seemed unheard of here. When the oncologist told Jim she was sorry they had "failed," Jim told her he did not appreciate her negative attitude. I know how broken his spirit was. Here were his doctors discussing his next procedure, yet doing so negatively without conveying any hope or optimism. About a week after this, Jim decided to meet with one of his fraternity friends, a lawyer, to talk about making a will.

In mid-December, we returned to the University of Wisconsin Hospital for several days of tests. Jim's cryopreserve autologous bone marrow harvest was scheduled for December 29. Then we returned to Minnesota for Christmas at home. Christmas of 1989 was hopeful once again—though Jim was plagued by a constant, nagging cough. He had experienced the same cough at Christmas of 1987 and in the summer of 1988. Jim's grandparents and Bryan came from Wausau to be with us for Christmas. Jim was especially proud when he saw how pleased his grandparents were with his aerial photos of their cottage. This would be the last Christmas we would have Jim with us.

Jim saw five patients on Dec. 27, the last full day he would spend in the practice he had self-started and would know success in within just four years. The following day we left for Madison.

Crosses to Bear

On December 29, 1989, Jim was admitted to the University of Wisconsin Hospital in Madison for his bone marrow harvest and cryopreservation. At this hospital we found outstanding care and genuine compassion. A few days after the harvest procedure, Jim received the cytoreductive salvage chemotherapy, which consisted of Ara-C, cisplatinum and dexamethasone. Al and I spent another New Year's Eve with Jim in the hospital. When he fell asleep, just before midnight, we returned to nearby Stoughton. The following day Al returned to Minnesota and I stayed on with Jim for another week's hospitalization. In his hospital room, before Al left, Jim had his dad give him a final short haircut—knowing that he would be losing his hair from the strong chemo he would be given. Jim had a beautiful head of hair and this wasn't an easy decision for him. He put it off until the very last minute.

Cycle I of this massive treatment of high-dose chemotherapy, begun in the first days of January, made Jim extremely ill and left him in excruciating pain. On one of these days he questioned, for the only time, the horrendous cross he had been given to bear. He said, "Mom, why must I suffer so? Am I so different from my brothers and sisters?" "No, Jim," I answered, "You are the most loving, caring child one could have. I don't know why this has happened. Just know that we will get through it." This was an extremely difficult day for Jim and so I stayed overnight at the hospital—sleeping on a cot in his room. A week later, I rented a car for our return trip home. Jim had endured the intense nausea of the chemo but the pounding, ever-present headaches were almost more than he could bear. I remember him saying, "Mom, don't go any slower than you have to!" This, in spite of my 75 mph speed—ten mph over the limit!

At home, although Jim pushed liquids constantly, the headaches remained. They completely incapacitated him. Only by lying in a prone position could he alleviate them somewhat. As soon as he attempted to stand, they would become unbearable and he would become dizzy and disoriented, with a ringing in his ears. On January 15, Jim tried to return to his practice but was able to see only one patient.

Not long after, Jim had to be hospitalized again at the University of Minnesota, this time for fungal infections. He would be plagued with these infections through both cycles of the massive chemotherapy, as the high doses of drugs destroyed his immunity to fight these infections. At this time Jim also began to notice the itching problem that would bother him months later. One of the resident students, who was making rounds with the doctor, blurted out, "Well, that's the Hodgkins, back again." I couldn't believe this resident student's audacity or license to say this. Once said, how can something like this be retracted?

Jim was also beginning to have more problems with the catheter implant, which had been placed in January of the previous year. Without the use of the implant, it was difficult to continually find blood vessels for drawing blood and receiving chemo treatments. It was especially crucial to have the use of this inlet for the upcoming bone marrow transplant, the daily blood draws it would require, and the intravenous port for necessary blood transfusions, antibiotics, and nutrition. So the doctors at the U of M tried surgery twice—to reposition the catheter in his chest. Both surgeries were unsuccessful.

We returned to Madison the end of January for Jim's second round of chemo to be given in February. Doctors at the University of Wisconsin Hospital were able to successfully reimplant the catheter—this time in the groin of his leg. Though I did not know it then, the doctors were aware of a tumor that was wrapped around Jim's aorta. Jim was hospitalized until February 7 when he and I drove back to Minnesota. I was about to begin a journey of my own.

In late January, before Jim and I left for Madison, I had noticed a kind of quirk or tenderness, at times, in my lower right pelvic area and wondered if it could be my appendix. As we walked out the door, I had asked Al to make an appointment for me with my doctor sometime in February. Soon after our return, however, I noticed that I could feel a definite lump that seemed to be getting appreciatively and considerably larger each day. And so, one week after our return, I called to make an appointment with my gynecologist. He saw me the same day, Thursday, February 15, and scheduled surgery for the following Monday. When he said he wanted to do a laparotomy, I knew this was serious. Jim had had the same procedure in January of 1986. When I walked into the house, Jim asked, "What is it, Mom?" It hurt so very much for him to hear the news because we both knew what it might mean. That evening Jim spiked a fever. Al was working late, as was his custom. So once again, Jim and I went to the Emergency Room at University Hospital. As Jim lay on one of the ER tables, receiving a blood transfusion, I lay on the one next to him. Silently we pondered the days ahead.

Two days later, on Saturday eve, Jim spiked yet another fever—this time caused by a resistant staph infection. Now, as I prepared for my surgery, Al assumed the role of caregiver, taking Jim to the University Hospital for admission.

My surgery, at Midway Hospital on the following Monday, February 19, revealed a malignant tumor that had broken through the wall of my colon. Surgeons removed the right half of my colon, the tumor, and nine lymph nodes, four of which were also malignant. When I asked about my prognosis, I was told it was 40-45 percent and that the first year's survival was the most crucial. Now I was sharing the same prognosis Jim had been given. Though I shared with the children the results of the surgery and my diagnosis, I don't believe I told them the prognosis. Naturally,

I was shocked at the severity of the diagnosis and the prognosis. But, it did not consume me; I was too concerned for Jim.

I was so happy when, five days later, I was able to cajole the doctor into an early discharge. Kathy told me later that as we walked into the University Hospital to visit Jim, I "sprinted" through the revolving door. I was just so happy to be able to reassure Jim by walking into his hospital room that Mom was doing fine. And although I was discharged at 99 lbs., I felt my usual energy and was anxious to be with Jim. I know this was not an easy time for him, worrying about both of us. During the five days of my own hospitalization, Al had had double duty, visiting both of us each day, in separate hospitals, all the while working full days.

On February 28, when Al was seeing Jim off by medical van to Madison, Jeanne was taking me to my post-surgical and oncology doctor appointments. Between my two appointments we drove to the hospital, hoping to see Jim before the medical van left. The medical van was pulling out of the hospital drive, just as we drove in. I felt tremendous relief, however, knowing Jim would soon be back under the care of Dr. Longo at the University of Wisconsin.

Two days later, after receiving the okay from my surgeon, Al and I drove to Madison. We were with Jim for the weekend and I scheduled a second-opinion visit with one of the oncologists at the University of Wisconsin Comprehensive Cancer Center. Their recommended protocol for my diagnosis was the same as I had received at home. On our return to Minnesota, I met with two doctors and made my choice of oncologist, Dr. Irving Lerner. Both he and my surgeon recommended that I begin my year of chemotherapy on March 19.

Jim's doctors spent most of March working to keep the candida infection under control and to free him of the staph infection so that he could begin the next round of high-dose chemo prior to the transplant. The hospital was also awaiting approval from Blue Cross/Blue Shield for the autologous bone marrow transplantation (BMT). They had given their approval earlier and then reversed their decision. I would learn later that pretransplant evaluation had revealed a large left mediastinal mass, involving the pericardium and extending out into the peripheral left lung. But, there had been shrinkage of these lesions prior to transplant.

During the second half of this month, when he did not have to be hospitalized and the insurance approval was being awaited, Jim stayed at his home-away-from-home with Kathy and her family. Because of his susceptibility to infection, their home had to be free of things such as pets, plants, and smoke. The plants and dog found temporary homes and Kathy gave up smoking.

Finally, afraid of awaiting the Blue Cross approval beyond when the doctors felt Jim was ready, we told them to go ahead and we would somehow manage the costs. The Blue Cross insurance coverage was then approved and the transplant surgery was scheduled for March 26.

The Last Battle

THOUGH WE KNEW THE BONE MARROW TRANSPLANT WAS a life-threatening procedure, we were certain that this would be the last battle in Jim's return to health. Once through it, we would return to happier lives. How could I think this beautiful child would not get well, while his family and peers matured?

During Jim's many hospitalizations, in addition to visiting, and administering to his needs, at his request, I read to him. It was a diversion for him and what he appreciated most. At the University of Minnesota, we read *The Power of Myth* (by Joseph Campbell) and *The Day the Universe Changed* (by James Burke). Now he requested the seven-volume series *Chronicles of Narnia* (by C. S. Lewis). These books had been favorites of his since his days at Our Lady Queen of Peace Elementary School in Madison, when one of the nuns had introduced him to them. Since Jim's books were back home, we borrowed the set that he had given to his niece, Terri, and this would be our almost-daily reading for the next six weeks. All of the reading was done through a mask. In fact, since March, when Jim returned to Madison, all of our hospital visits required mask, gloves, gown and booties. That included hugs and kisses.

The preparative regimen of autologous bone marrow transplantation began. It consisted of high dose Thiotepa and Etoposide for three consecutive days. This was followed by the infusion of Jim's previously cryopreserved bone marrow.

During this week before Jim's transplant, I had to be back in the Twin Cities to begin my own chemotherapy. The initial round was one week of daily treatment of Fluorouracil (5FU). Thereafter, 5FU would be given by injection every Monday for one year. I also took oral doses of a new experimental drug, Levamisole. These were taken every eight hours for three days, every other week. Levamisole had been pioneered, as a treatment for colon cancer, at the University of Wisconsin Comprehensive Cancer Center.

On the following Monday, March 26, I drove to Madison to be with Jim. The bone marrow transplant was accomplished that day and his post transplant course began. Our readings helped take Jim's mind off his growing discomfort. But as the ravages of the pre-transplant chemo did their work, Jim suffered terribly for weeks. In addition to not being able to eat, he could not swallow without pain. The tissues, from his mouth down, had been literally "burned out" and the skin of his buttocks resembled dry, red leather—which had to be moisturized and lubricated constantly. The six-week period following the bone marrow transplantation required support with intravenous antibiotics, total parenteral nutrition (TPN), and transfusions of red blood cells and platelets. This was a period of profound anemia and mucositis. Jim's pain was physical; mine was secondary—that of a mother seeing her son having to endure all this. I wondered how other people could choose to treat their bodies with disrespect. Jim had done nothing to bring about these atrocities to his body.

Toward the end of the week, I had to make a quick trip back home, as I was beginning to feel the minor side effects of my daily chemo—namely, mouth sores and cold sores. I saw my oncologist in Minnesota and received the needed medication for this problem.

Then, after my Monday treatment, I returned again to Madison, to be with Jim on his 32nd birthday—April 5. It was not a joyful birthday for him, though it was a grateful one, I think. Jeanne sent him a journal; and, Steve, a cheerful, jade, Members-Only jacket. Kathy, Joan Janssen, and I visited with him, and the nurses and doctors did their best to make the day special. When I gave him the portable CD player from Al and me, Jim thought it was too "spendy." In all the months he would be hospitalized there,

Jim would ask for only one thing: two pictures to hang on the wall of this very sterile room—one of our family and one of our Wisconsin lake cottage. "It's one of my favorite places," he often said. Over the years, I believe his heart had bonded with the lake.

As my role of caretaker was compromised with my diagnosis and treatment, Kathy, and our friends, Joan and Ron Janssen and Rose and Dale McCutcheon stepped in to help. Kathy visited Jim when I was unable to be there, as did Joan and Dale. Before the transplant, when Jim had permission to leave the hospital, both couples invited Jim and me over to their homes for dinners and visits. In late April and early May, as his blood counts continued to build, he was able to leave the hospital for outings. Both Joan and Dale took Jim out for drives, walks, and visits to the Arboretum.

Jim had always been concerned about receiving blood transfusions and, because Jim and I were the same blood type, I had offered in December to gain a little weight and be a donor for Jim. Dr. Longo, however, had discouraged my doing so. He had said, "As Jim's principal caregiver, you must maintain your strength for that." There were, also, many other cross-matches for this type of donor. One who did give blood was Ron Janssen. Ron was a runner and in good physical condition and Jim felt very good about receiving blood from him. During one of his trying days following the transplant, when Jim needed blood, he showed his ever-present sense of humor—which he maintained through all these terrible ordeals. He asked the nurse if she could tell him whether the transfusion he was receiving was from Ron. She, of course, answered, "No." Jim replied, "Well, if I get up tomorrow morning and want to run seven miles, I'll know it was Ron's blood!"

Because of my treatments and also because I still had to run the practice, there were times when I could not be in Madison every day. To maintain the practice, both for the welfare of the patients and for Jim's return, we had engaged a dentist, part-time. When I wasn't there to assist, I hired temporaries for both hygiene and assisting. Jeanne retrieved phone messages daily and scheduled our patients for us.

When I couldn't be with Jim during the week, Al and I would go for the weekends. Many times Steve, Jeanne, and Jim's niece, Amanda, would accompany us. One weekend, Steve had just begun his first job after graduating from the University of Minnesota School of Engineering. A mechanical engineer, he had started as a development engineer with Pfizer's American Medical Systems, designing urological implants for both incontinence and impotence. Kathy remembers Steve being a bit embarrassed and uncomfortable about explaining his first project to his siblings. But Jim was enjoying it "big-time," and, literally "bursting" to tell Kathy the news.

In April, we all went down for two weekends—my birthday and Easter. Bryan came from Wausau with my parents, and the Lukens "hotel" provided accommodations. When we could not be there, we had always called Jim, daily. First, we would speak to the unit nurse and learn Jim's daily blood counts. They were rising slowly but steadily, and, according to expectations. Then the nurse would transfer us to Jim's room. If his voice never seemed very "up," we could understand why but we always had a good, lengthy conversation anyway. Only later did we learn the effects of his monitored, self-administered morphine. One day, weeks later, Jim seemed extra happy and told Kathy, "Mom and Dad called." "They've been doing that every night," she told her surprised brother. The morphine had kept him from remembering our calls.

When we went for the Mother's Day weekend, we had a pleasant surprise. Jim had been discharged that day to Kathy and Gary's home. When we had visited him in his hospital room we had to be masked and, when he left his room for our in-hospital walks, this was reversed and he had to mask. Therefore, this was a happy, happy weekend—the first time in months we could exchange kisses and hugs without all the isolation encumbrances of masks, gown, and gloves. My mother and father came from Wausau with my brother, Ed, and sister-in-law, Corrine. So I was able to be with Mother, also, on Mothers' Day. We had a joyful weekend and on Saturday evening played *Life Stories.* This game provided an evening of laughter, reminiscing, and revelations. In his answers to questions, we learned that Jim considered all of his birthdays as "special" and that his favorite toys and pastimes included his green truck, the stilts his father made for him, his walkie-talkies, and climbing the tree in Wausau to see the horses on the hill below our land. Another question, however, evoked an answer which, in retrospect, is most poignant. To, "Where would you live if you could live anywhere?" Jim replied, "Here . . . with my family."

The following week, Jim began walking with Kathy, driving his car, and going to Mass with Kathy. On their afternoon or evening walks, they would critique neighboring homes, gardens and landscaping. And then, by Jim's choice, they would end their walks in a nearby cemetery, where she knew he sometimes walked alone. And, she tried not to think too much of it at the time.

Kathy also recalls the many good times she and Jim had together during the weeks he stayed at their home. One day Kathy, who was known to bring surprises home from garage sales, returned from a flea market with a bag of potatoes. Gary and Jim sighed with relief. This was something they could actually use—but, *fifty pounds* of potatoes? On another occasion, after Jim had cooked one of his pasta dinners for them, she was cleaning up in their makeshift kitchen. (The restoration of this room in their Victorian home had been suspended for the six months that Jim was with them on-and-off.) She had just had a new perm and a very short haircut, and she heard Jim's voice from the living room, "Is there a boy in our kitchen?"

On the weekend following, when we returned to Stoughton, Jim had made a pasta dinner for all of us on Friday as Kathy and I were planning our second 17-mile Syttende Mai walk the next morning. And, as Jim's recuperation was proceeding nicely, we began to plan ahead for a gathering at the cottage in June—to celebrate Jim's grandparents' 65th wedding anniversary and our 40th. We also began thinking ahead to his return home on July 4—after the required 100-day stay within 100 miles of the transplant site.

Another Limbo

THEN, IN ONE OF OUR PHONE CONVERSATIONS ON MAY 24, I heard Jim cough—the same ominous cough that had plagued him at the time of his recurrence in December of 1989. He had mentioned it to the doctors and, when I was with him the following week for his weekly check-up at the Clinic, they said they felt it was an infection of some kind—as the nodules, which appeared on the x-ray, seemed hollow.

Thus began another time of Limbo for us. I say for us; it was, of course, both physically and mentally difficult for Jim. For us, it was mental and emotional, as we hurt so for what was happening to our son and for being so limited in helping him through these ordeals.

A month of searching, testing and waiting began. Jim's lungs were bronchoscoped, biopsied, and lavaged. When I asked Jim if we should cancel the June party at the cottage, he insisted we proceed; his doctors and nurses had planned to be there with him. We also talked of his return to his practice and he said he wanted to hire an assistant so that I would be free to concentrate on marketing and managing the office.

The following weekend was spent at the cottage. Bryan, and Jeanne and Amanda, came to help Jim's grandparents and Al and me in a work weekend of raking, cleaning and readying for the June 16 party. My mother had fractured her pelvis the previous week and, after spending a few days with my mother and dad, I returned to Madison to visit Jim.

Jim enjoyed the anniversary observance on Saturday—a Mass, dinner and open house. It could not have been easy for him, as

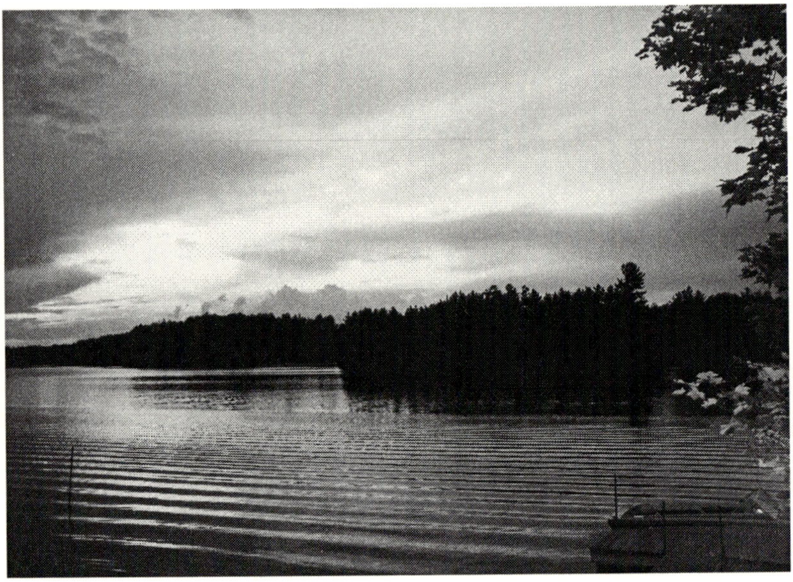

Lake Somo, at sunset. Jim was finally able to return to one of his favorite places.

both he and we were wondering about the cough. But, visiting with relatives and friends he had not seen for some time was a good diversion for him and I think he truly found pleasure in this. At day's end, someone built a campfire in the firepit on the lakeshore. Most of the guests had left and Jim borrowed someone's guitar. Around the campfire, with the family gathered, he played and sang with all of us. To this day, I would like to share the lakeside campfires, but find I cannot. I can only remember that one. Only when

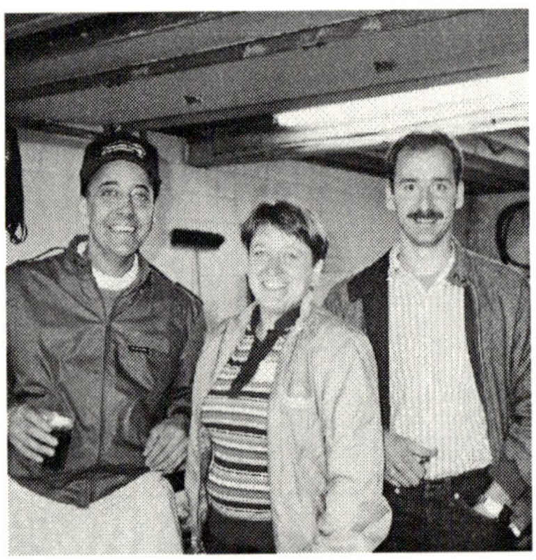

Jim with sister, Jeanne, and brother, Steve, at the double anniversary celebration for his parents and grandparents—at their Tomahawk cottage. June 16, 1990

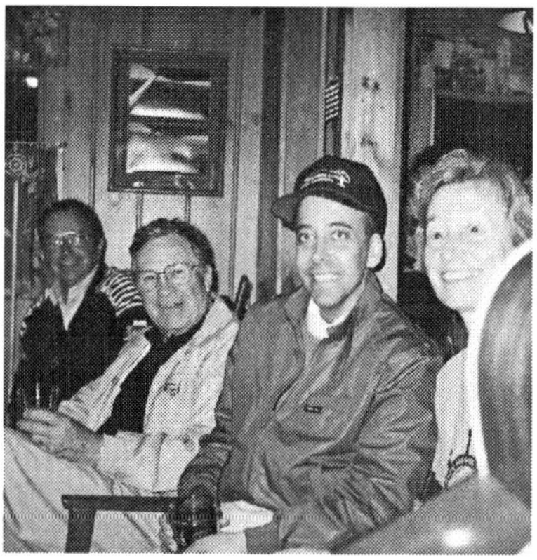

In the evening, after some 100 guests had departed, Jim relaxed with his Dad, his uncle, Jim Madden, and myself—before playing the guitar at a lakeside campfire.

it is subdued, with the immediate family present, or when it is functional, such as for roasting marshmallows, can I bring myself to partake. Jim's doctors and nurses did not come; everyone had a reason, of course. Did they, in fact, already know what would soon be their bad news for us?

The day following the anniversaries was Fathers' Day, and, after observing that occasion and taking some pictures, Kathy and

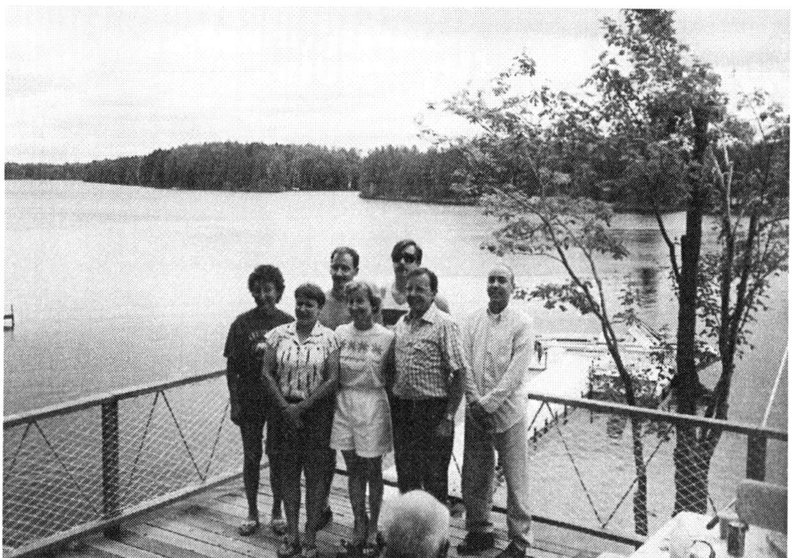

The following day, Fathers' Day, our last family picture! A week later, on June 26, Jim and we would be told by his doctors that the Hodgkin's had returned and he had only weeks to live!

Gary left for Minocqua, Wisconsin to tour a new time-share and claim their prize of a Lincoln or a radio. Instead, they returned as new time-share owners, and Jim couldn't believe they had let themselves be talked into doing such a thing! But, he did enjoy the unbelief and the teasing he could give them on their return trip to Madison. And we returned to the Twin Cities for me to catch up with my work at the practice.

A week later, Tuesday, June 26, the call came. It was the most awful news of our life. It was one of Jim's doctors, Dr. Hong. He said, "I just had a very saddened talk with Jim." I knew immediately what those words meant. And, I remember that sentence—word for word. The Hodgkin's had returned and there was no other treatment to pursue. Jim had wanted him to make the call to us. Then we spoke to Jim. Again, so limited! What does one say to a son when he has been told he will soon die? Again, he received the terrible news alone. But, this was so much worse, and this time we were miles and hours apart.

I asked the doctor if we couldn't find another way to lick this. He said, "No." Over the period of observation, Jim's mediastinal lesions had increased in size and new lesions had developed. I asked how long Jim might live. His answer was chilling: "Several weeks. We will do all we can to make him comfortable." My immediate thought was that, if he didn't say a couple of months, it will only be about seven weeks. That was exactly what it would be. My other reaction was, "Why, oh why, did he tell Jim this when we couldn't be there with him?" Did Jim perhaps suspect or know and then ask the doctor outright? It just hurt so to know he was alone.

After we'd spoken with Jim, we immediately called Kathy and she and Gary went to the hospital to be with Jim. We left early the next morning, and visited and cried with Jim. I do not know exactly what we spoke of. Those minutes are foggy in my memory. Al drove home to pick up our new van and I drove Jim's car home a few days later when I came home for my chemo treatment. Jeanne and Amanda returned to Madison with us and, after we'd gone through the mechanics of Jim's discharge, we stayed with Kathy and her family overnight. It was extremely hot and, without air-conditioning, Jim needed to be on oxygen for the first time.

Then, on July 5, the day that was to have been Jim's triumphant return home—100 days after his transplant—we were, instead, bringing our son home to die.

At Home

WHEN JIM WAS HOME, WE CONTACTED NEW ENGLAND Critical Care for assistance in setting up needed supplies and equipment. With air conditioning in our home, he would not need, nor would he even think of using, oxygen at first. It was only a backup and we would, of course, take it with us for our planned week at the cottage.

Because the doctors considered Jim to be moderately malnourished, he received total parenteral nutrition (TPN) by intravenous feeding. In addition, I kept a daily record of the calories he consumed in his meals and snacks. As soon as we had a daily routine established, we prepared to go to the cottage—which was Jim's first desire. The nurses set us up with all of the necessary materials, along with a referral to the Lincoln County Visiting Nurses, should we need them.

We loaded our new van and took off for the cottage. Jeanne and Amanda went with us. Bryan, along with Jim's grandparents, joined us there. It was to be for about a week, and the trip went well—much better than the return trip from Madison had been. In retrospect, I wish we had gone a few weeks later; I think Jim would have been able to enjoy it more. This first week, he was still on "the pole." His total parenteral nutrition (TPN), and the necessary antibiotics were all taken intravenously. It just seemed he was almost always "hooked up" and had so little freedom to enjoy his time there. In addition, he did not feel very well. I remember the nights, especially, being difficult for him; neither he nor I slept well and he had to call me often during the night. I remember, also, mentally listing which of Jim's friends, and which of

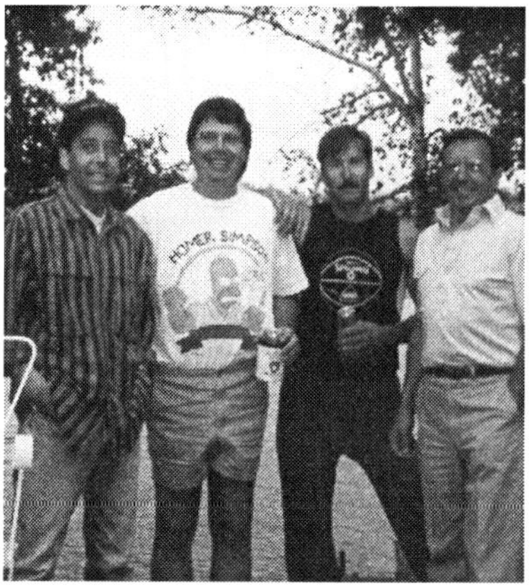

One of Jim's wishes was for a return to the cottage. From the cottage, we took a day trip to the home of Jim's aunt and uncle at Manitowish Waters, Wisconsin—as his cousin, John, was visiting from Denver. Jim; cousin, John; brother, Bryan; and Dad

our friends and relatives, were nurses and might be available to help with night duty once we were back home. None of this was necessary. When we returned home, Jim began to feel much better. And halcion allowed him to sleep better. Jim never, ever, did expect or ask anything of anyone that they didn't offer on their own and want to do for him.

Jim's grandparents were with us at the cottage. This would be the last visit they would have with their grandson. During the week, one of Jim's cousins from Colorado was visiting Jim's aunt and uncle in Manitowish Waters. By this time, we had called the doctor and had received permission to shed some of the prescribed IV treatment. So we took a day trip to our relatives, the Maddens, at their lake home in northern Wisconsin. I still find it amazing, when I look at a picture taken that day, to see Jim with a smile on his face. I marvel at his spirit and strength.

When I came across that picture, after Jim's death, I remembered a favorite poem of his. Though I do not recall how it came to be in his possession,

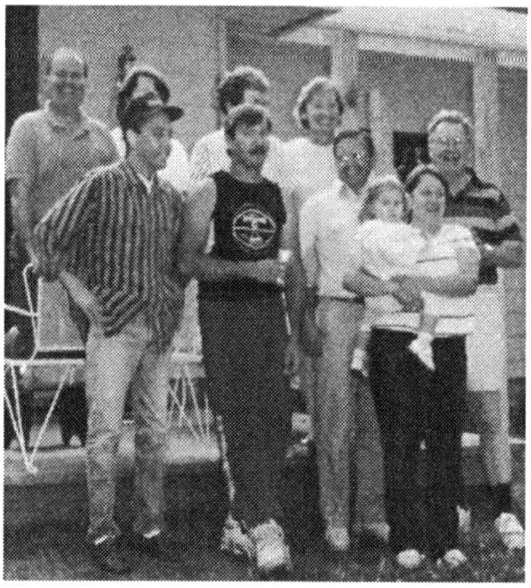

Another picture with family and friends—though smiling on the outside, we're crying on the inside.

I recall his having it shortly after his original diagnosis. I remember, too, his sending and sharing it with someone in need of a smile. I found it and quote it here:

A Smile to Wish You Well

There's a secret knack to living
that can shorten every mile.
When the load gets too oppressive,
you can lighten it with a smile.
When your world crowds in about you,
what can cheer you for a while?
The finest therapy you know,
the simplest one—a smile!

When troubles come to try us,
to irritate or rile,
it's easy to explode or weep
but it's better far to smile.
If you laugh, the world laughs with you,
and admires your grace and style.
Things have a way of working out,
so help them along with a smile!

Back home from the cottage, things settled into a routine. We were living one precious day at a time. Jim was no longer on any IV and his "old" appetite returned. Jim had two appointments with my oncologist, Dr. Irving Lerner. And because he was doing so much better, I even hoped that on his second visit to Dr. Lerner, a chest x-ray would reveal the tumor to be miraculously shrinking. During this time, too, the fingernails that Jim had lost to the chemo began to grow back. When Jim died, he had new growth of both hair and fingernails.

Steve, Jeanne, and Amanda visited almost every day, and Jim's friends from Hill-Murray High School, along with their wives and card-club friends, came regularly, too. They recommended videos that would give us some laughter therapy. One friend brought her Mr. Juice machine and something like fifty pounds of carrots. Jim would choose the juice combinations he would like and we hoped this, too, would help. The last time Jim drove his car, which he had just purchased in September of 1989 from his grandparents, was about two weeks before his death. He went to dinner at the home of his Hill-Murray friends, Jim and Kathy Miettunen—with the oxygen tanks packed in the trunk. On another day, Jim took Steve's newly purchased 1966 Corvette out for a drive, sitting very proudly behind the wheel of his brother's new toy.

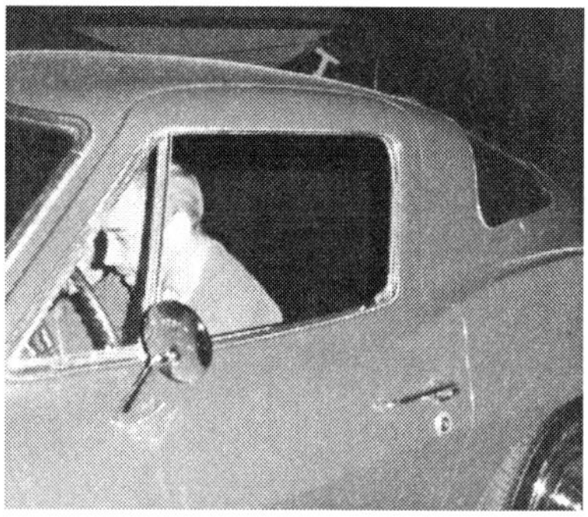

Just weeks before Jim's death, he was able to drive his brother Steve's newly acquired 1966 Corvette.

So happy for his brother, Jim seemed to really enjoy the experience.

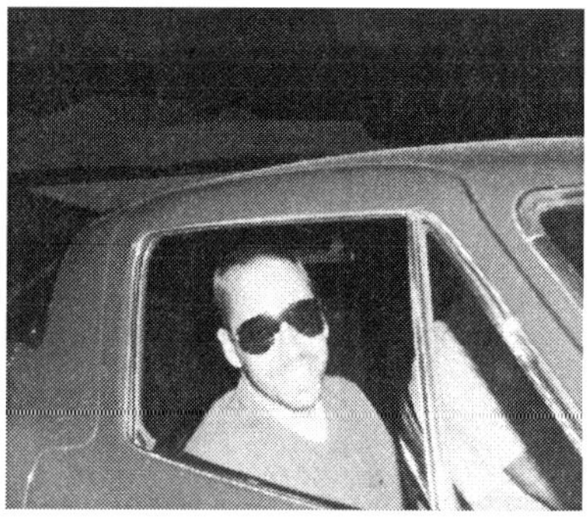

During this time, one of the symptoms that bothered Jim most was a constant itching on his whole body—which he experienced the whole seven weeks at home. Hydroxyzine medication did not even give him much relief. He always appreciated getting a backrub as that seemed to distract enough from the symptom to get some relief. During the day I did this for him. But my arms are not my strongest appendage and I didn't have much endurance. So it was a real treat for Jim when Al, Jeanne, Steve, or one of his visiting Hill-Murray friends took over for me. Jeanne remembers that many times when she gave him a backrub, he was wearing his windsurfing T-shirt. He had earned the shirt years before, when a dental-friend couple took him windsurfing for the first time. He'd been caught out on the water without enough wind to return and had to paddle the board back in. Jeanne would ask for this shirt after Jim's death.

Once again, on Jim's request, we tried finding a book that I could read to him; none proved apropos. *The Chronicles of Narnia,* read in the hospital, would be the last. And that, at times, had been most difficult, as there were passages—with references to dying—that we had both found very poignant at the time. Unsuccessful at books, we turned to one of Jim's favorite games, Trivial Pursuit. He and I played that game for hours nearly every day. Over the weeks, keeping score, he won more than two-thirds of the time, beating me in all categories.

There are many should-have's. Why didn't I play the piano? Jim especially liked one of my old recital pieces; it was one the children had always requested. Yet, it seemed we did all we could and filled every hour.

Meanwhile, Jim's practice continued with the same dentist we had hired in January, but only on days she could be there and I could hire an assistant. I rarely went in to the Eden Prairie office during these weeks. Al, whose office was in Bloomington, brought home the mail so that I could pay bills and keep up with insurance claims and billing. I either had the telephone calls forwarded or retrieved messages from home at convenient times.

Jim always watched the morning news shows, and this is when I would do the office work in an adjoining room. During this time, also, Jim must have penned his words for his will. For, after his death, I would find the paper, dated July 26. One of the most difficult tasks I faced during those weeks was taking Jim to his attorney's office to sign his will—such a finality for a young man, our son. In it he voiced his wish that his beneficiaries would donate ten percent of their inheritance to their favorite charity—"in memory of me and my priorities, goals and aspirations." Jim, for his part, left $6,000 to three charities: The American Cancer Society, The United Fund, and the Christian Children's Fund. The first two charities were most grateful in acknowledging Jim's bequests. The United Fund, after coming to our home to visit with us and learn about Jim, set up an endowment in his memory. We never heard from the third charity.

Following our daily routines, I would prepare the evening dinners which Jim helped plan. It was so encouraging to see him enjoying meals once again. As we awaited Al for dinner, we would watch "Bill Cosby"—another exercise in laughter. In the evenings after dinner, if we were not visiting with Jim's family or friends who stopped by, Jim, Al and I might watch a rented video; then, always, the 10:00 news and "Cheers." By this time, Jim used oxygen occasionally during the day and, always, at night. We attached the long plastic tubing to the oxygen machine in the living room so that Jim wouldn't hear the noise of the machine in his bedroom. Then Al carried the tubing as the three of us walked down the hall to the bedrooms.

Another of our last outings was one last trip to the hospital—Midway, this time. As an outpatient, the implanted catheter that Jim had lived with for nineteen months was removed.

We continued thus until early August when Jim reluctantly decided he would call Hospice, as the doctors and discharging staff had recommended. It was one thing Aware Gold didn't cover and this bothered Jim; he was still on the old austerity program. Though we probably only needed about seven visits from St. Joseph's Hospice, they were wonderful to us. Every single one of the nurses who came out was most compassionate and caring. When the Hospice social worker asked if he was afraid of dying, Jim said, "No, but it hurts when I see my Mom cry." At this time, Jim had so little control over things that were happening in his life and I wanted him to have control over things he could. So I did not bring up the subject of dying. I did not want to hurt him with my tears that would most surely come. I managed only to try and confirm that he still favored cremation. It still seemed so; though now he wondered if one was not polluting the atmosphere in the process of cremation. One Hospice nurse, Mary, asked Jim what she could do for him and he mentioned the itching. She had been trained as a masseuse, and she gave him an hour-long, full-body massage, as he sat in the recliner chair, which had by now become his.

I cannot imagine the thoughts Jim had to endure each day. Yet, faced with his own death, he was still most empathetic about others. Joan Janssen recalls Jim's concern at this time for Angie, Joan and Ron's granddaughter who was facing a medical concern that summer.

Jim's last outing, five days before he died, was a trip to the home of his Hill-Murray friends, Bill and Helen Hutton, for a cook-out get-together with the whole Hill-Murray and card club group. One of Jim's friends picked him up and he told her that, although he did not really feel up to going, he thought Mom and Dad needed a few hours. Later, when they called to tell us that Jim was ready to go home, he told them that he was glad he had come; he had a really good time. He was, also, looking forward to another trip to the cottage the following weekend.

"I Wish, I Wish . . ."

TO RECOUNT JIM'S LAST THREE DAYS, I RELIVE, AS I DO so many times, the agony. This will ever after be my mark of time: before Jim's death, after Jim's death.

On Thursday, Jim said he thought it would be better if we waited until Friday to go to the cottage. On Friday, it became another decision.

Every day, during his last seven weeks at home, Jim had gotten out of bed, dressed for the day, and retired with us in the late evening. Friday, August 10, would be different. All day he tried desperately to feel better, to get up, to eat. He said to me, "I have to eat to keep up my strength." On the nurses prodding, Jim finally consented to having a hospital bed delivered. And, though she also ordered a hospital-type chair, he would have nothing to do with it! Dad's reclining chair was just fine. Jim never rallied much that day. Around dinnertime, we called Hospice for a nurse to visit. When she arrived, she asked if we had called a priest. Because we had not, she called for us—both St. Patrick's in Edina, Jim's home parish, and St. Mary of the Lake in White Bear Lake. Father Mike Krenik from St. Pat's was the first to return our call. He said he would come out immediately. It's about a 30-mile drive and he arrived sometime after 10 P.M. Steve and Jeanne were with us, and Father Mike gave Jim the Sacrament of the Sick. Before beginning, he explained, "Now you know, Jim, this is not considered the Last Sacrament; it's meant to be a blessing for the sick." Still true to his reputation for good humor, Jim quipped, "Oh, don't worry, Father—I plan on waking up tomorrow morning." He was still giving us a good laugh, still not allowing himself any self-pity.

Saturday was another day in bed. Already on twelve medications, Jim had begun using morphine during the night. He was not feeling very well and was allowed morphine every four hours. At one stretch he was able to manage for twelve hours without it; another time he could only manage for two hours. Father Roger Pierre, our priest from St. Mary's, had called the previous night shortly after Father Mike had. On Saturday morning he came to visit and said a prayer for all of us: Jim, Al, Jeanne, Steve, and me. In the afternoon, a Hill-Murray friend, Jim Miettunen, called and stopped by; but around dinnertime, Jim asked to rest.

Sunday was to be our last day with our dear Jim. We had called Kathy and Bryan the day before to tell them that Jim was not doing well and that we would not see them in Wisconsin that weekend, as planned. When Al and I went to 7:30 Mass that morning, Father Roger related in his homily that he had visited the home of a family whose young son, a dentist, was dying of cancer. I was shocked when I heard these words spoken aloud. I don't believe I had allowed myself to believe this was happening. Now, this made it a harsh reality.

On Sunday, though his blood work revealed normal counts for white blood cells and platelets, Jim began having problems with nosebleeds. So Al and Jeanne went to pick up some Vitamin K—prescribed by the Hospice nurse. Jeanne remembers being apprehensive when the pharmacy gave them only a small number of pills. (And she had previously wondered why it was so imperative that Father Mike drive over so late on Friday evening.) We were still not ready for Jim to leave us. But Jeanne did ask Craig to pick up little Amanda earlier on Sunday afternoon so that she could stay later into the evening. I think we knew, though we never really wanted to admit it or believe it, that Jim was getting nearer the end. When Steve left Sunday evening, something he said led me to believe that he had not yet accepted the thought that Jim would die; he still felt Jim would get better. We all just "hoped" for a miracle so much—still believing it would happen. Sometimes you cannot believe what you see, you have to believe what you feel.

I think Jim did know the end was approaching. At bedtime, he asked me to get Al because he wanted to talk to us about something. It turned out to be a private, medical matter—Jim still the gentleman, still the professional! After Al said good-night to Jim, I asked Jim if he wanted me to stay with him. "Yes, Mom," he said. And so I did. We held hands as he dropped off to sleep and our love passed between us. I was alone with my thoughts until sometime after midnight, when Al awoke and said he would sit with Jim. Al thought I should try to get some rest. Soon after, Al called me to say Jim had become restless. While we were both sitting bedside with him, Jim suddenly sat up, pulled the oxygen tube from his nostrils, and said, "I wish, I wish . . . it doesn't matter." In our attempts to quiet his fears and replace the oxygen tube, we don't remember if we asked him what he meant. Those were to be Jim's last words. I shall wonder, forever, what he meant!

We were sitting alongside Jim when he died. It was about 5:30 A.M. on Monday morning, August 13, 1990. Life had left our beautiful, always caring, fun-loving son.

When we realized there was no pulse, we called Hospice and Jim's brothers and sisters. Jeanne and Steve came immediately to share our loss as we tried to support each other. The Hospice nurse and Father Roger came, also. Father Roger again gave us spiritual support and both he and the Hospice nurse helped us with the necessary decision-making. Bryan and Kathy and Gary arrived from Wisconsin the following day, and it was good to have everyone present in the difficult days that followed. When the Lukens grandchildren arrived they put together the photos of Jim for the picture boards for the funeral. That was something I could not have managed myself.

I cannot find the words to express the awful feeling of seeing our son carried out of our home on a mortician's gurney. Jim would never return—to bound up the steps, saying, "Mom, I'm home." I was grateful the mortician did not arrive until 9:30; that gave me another few short hours to sit with Jim. Death, to the touch, is not only still, quiet, and cold—but hard! When Jim's spirit left his body, it took his softness with it.

After Jim died, I found some writing he had done during his last weeks at home. Here are two of the entries:

My fingers don't work as they once did.
To my grandparents I leave my eternal
thanks for their role in shaping my parents.

I've never been much good at keeping
a journal, and that is certainly not what
this is. This is an emotional thanksgiving.
I thought of all the things for which I was
thankful, but I knew if I got into those
sorts of things I would start crying—so I
didn't say anything. Now I wish I had,
so I'm writing it here. I am blessed with
a family that has always loved me and that
always will. In addition to family, I have
friends who also give me compassion,
courage, and prayers. I never feel alone;
and I am thankful.

Letters to Jim

THIS JOURNAL TO OUR SON EVOLVED AS I FELT THE NEED to share some of my days' thoughts with Jim. On especially sad or joyful days, when I wanted so very much to talk with him, I was compelled to write my feelings. Putting these thoughts on paper seemed to bring me comfort and a measure of healing. It was, I believe, a kind of therapy.

We write to externalize—to put into words our thoughts and feelings. In telling our story, we release the pain. We may do it first for ourselves and, later, to share with others. It becomes a way to handle and to heal.

This same feeling of comfort and healing is repeated in the opportunities Al and I have taken to travel in the footsteps of Jim—to travel to places he'd visited and we had not, to frequent being in locales where he was most happy. In his physical absence, I find a need for connections and so I try to keep him alive, for myself, any way I can. In addition to frequenting places he enjoyed, we grow the roses he grew, listen to his CD's, and wear some of his items of clothing. In addition, I buy special remembering gifts at Jim's birthday time and at Christmas. These serve as physical reminders and memory joggers. I seem, also, to have a need for more music and flowers in my life.

There are so many things I wish I could share with Jim. In my genealogy work, when we have a really good find, he would have shared my excitement. It was Jim who first asked for pictures of his grandparents and who looked for our family name in different sources such as the Sigma Chi directory and the phone book. In looking at our ancestral tree, he and I often spoke of the longevity in our families. He said he thought when we approached our nineties, it would be o.k. to begin sitting in our rocking chairs.

Not a day passes without my thinking of Jim. I wish we had him with us still, in place of only memories. He has left only good thoughts and we have only these memories to sustain us. Please gift us with your remembering, also.

November 14, 1990

Dear Jim,

Copies of your will were sent to your beneficiaries on Oct. 8. And, as your siblings were reading these instruments of sadness, Grandma lay unconscious in St. Mary's Hospital—following a massive stroke just four days after her surgery for a broken hip. She died on October 11, and now she and you are together in Heaven. Are you and she playing cards together? Grandpa is devastated; and, my grief for you is so recent and so intense that I am numbed.

If your siblings don't speak of you often, I wonder about how they are handling their grief. Kathy has her family; Jeanne lives close and so we see her and speak of you. Steve has a sadness in his eyes so much of the time. In addition to losing a brother, he has lost his best friend. I did recently learn that he speaks of you in conversation with his peers and yours. Bryan is more miles away and I don't see his tears. But he called one night, sometime after receiving his copy of the will, and broke down and sobbed uncontrollably—almost unable to speak. We were glad he knew he could call us and share his feelings. I know we all handle our grief differently, but we must deal with it in some manner and help each other cry.

Love,

Mom

Christmas 1990

Dear Jim,

Our first Christmas without you! How can people still wish us a "Merry Christmas"? On Friday we drove to Wausau to pick up Grandpa so that he could spend Christmas with us. This is a most difficult holiday for him, too. We spent Christmas Eve at home, and then, after Mass on Christmas morning, we all drove to Madison to spend the day with Kathy, Gary, and family. At Mass,

I found I could not sing any of the Christmas carols; this used to be a beautiful part of my Mass. I could only remember your being with us last year.

Even more astounding than my not being able to sing is the fact that Dad can no longer whistle. He was attempting to teach Amanda how and found he could not! Our lives are so changed.

Love,
Mom

December 28, 1990

Dear Jim,

In the darkness and quiet of this winter season, I think the rest of our lives will be winter. I feel we will never laugh again. I don't plan for fun and laughter. When we do experience joy and laughter, however, it feels so very good. Your godchild, Amanda, is with us often as we care for her to help out Jeanne. This little two-year-old is a real blessing. Always cheerful, she brings joy and smiles to our life. Late this afternoon we took her tobogganing on the golf course hill behind our house (one of your old pastimes). In winter's early dusk, as we were pulling her on the toboggan back to the house, she quietly sang the whole way home, "Twinkle, twinkle, little star." It lifted us to the point of tears!

Love,
Mom

February 25, 1991

Dear Jim,

Today I had my last chemotherapy treatment. How I wish you could have celebrated it with me. The oncology nurses gave me a china rose with a butterfly alighting on it and Dr. Lerner told me I'd been a brick! Is that a compliment? When Dad lost his job a week after your funeral, he took me to my weekly chemo appointments and I really appreciated that. After your death, on the evening of my chemo treatments, I found I felt tired—something I hadn't noticed when you were here. I believe you build your strength from the people with whom you surround yourself. And, you were my strength—"the wind beneath my wings."

Love,

Mom

May 17, 1991

Dear Jim,

Just a year ago today we began our last happy weekend as we came to Madison to see you in your recuperation period at Kathy and Gary's home. You cooked dinner for us (a shrimp rotini casserole) to prepare Kathy and me for our 17-mile Syttende Mai walk on Saturday morning. And it will be a year next Thursday, when I called to talk to you, that I heard the awful, ominous cough—the same as you had had in November and December of 1989. Then followed a month of hoping the spots found in your lungs would prove to be an infection, as the doctors had said.

My heart is heavy; my tears won't stop. I miss you so. Both your dreams and ours were shattered.

Love,

Mom

May 24, 1991

Dear Jim,

Today Jeanne told us that Amanda has been making calls to you on her toy phone. How I wish she could be calling you at 942-0341, on her mother's real phone.

Love,

Mom

June 1, 1991

Dear Jim,

Today we sold your practice and we couldn't really feel very happy. All of your dedication and success—sold for about half its present worth, only $30,000. But it was the best we could do—eleven months of trying (after you had put it in real estate hands last July). By now, you would have built it to at least three times that value.

But, it was time. For these past eleven months, I have been both managing the practice and assisting, with the help of dentists we have hired. It will seem different not making the drive to Eden Prairie each day, and I shall miss the company and support I've received from your patients.

Then we went to a Mass we had said for you at St. Patrick's in Edina—the church to which you belonged and where, as a tenor, you had sung in the choir. Steve, Shelly, and Kurt came, too. Afterwards we took them out for pizza. We missed you! Steve was on a roll, laughwise. It was like mealtime when you and he would be here for dinner and we'd all roar in laughter—as the two of you were such humorous complements to each other.

Love,
Mom

June 16, 1991

Dear Jim,

A year ago today was the last day spent together with hope. As I look at the family picture of us on that Father's Day (the day after the anniversary party), you look so happy—your usual confident self. Oh, how much I hurt!

This year, we planted a weeping willow tree down by the lake—in memory of you and your grandmother. We know you are happy in each other's company and I feel you are with us in spirit. Just after Saturday's planting session, and following a few drops of rain, there appeared in the sky a beautiful rainbow—a reminder of our beautiful, colorful days when you were with us.

We love you,
Mom

June 25, 1991

Dear Jim,

This Tuesday, a year ago, was one of the three saddest days of my life. We received a phone call in the evening from Dr. Hong. He said, "I just had a very saddened conversation with Jim, in which I had to tell him the Hodgkin's had returned (as nodules in the lung), and there is no more treatment we can give." We had hoped for the past month that this was an infection.

The disbelief and pain were, and are, unbearable. But why did he have to tell you this when you were alone. Couldn't he have waited until we came for the weekend? Or did you ask?

Then when we spoke to you, the few words we found were so inadequate. In our absence, I'm thankful that Kathy and Gary were able to respond to our call for help and go directly to the hospital to be with you. After packing our suitcases it was so long awaiting our morning departure, and it would be the longest trip we'd ever taken to Madison.

I love you,
Mom

Be with me with your loving spirit always.

June 27, 1991

Dear Jim,

Today I read a note you had penned to your Master Card company two days after being told you had "weeks to live." And *yet,* your usual humor was present! In the note you told them to "consider the account closed" and that you were "going with a no-annual-fee card."

How does one actually laugh and cry at the same time?

Love,
Mom

July 3, 1991

Dear Jim,

Driving to Wausau for your cousin Maria's wedding and to visit your remains at the Mausoleum Chapel, I can only think of a year ago. We were going home with you from Kathy and Gary's home in Stoughton. The long-awaited 100 days after your bone marrow transplant and we were going home—for you to die! We had been planning, after 100 days, to bring you home to recuperate and resume your life and your practice. It was to have been a glorious long-awaited return! What poor, rotten luck! Our life will never be the same, nor will we. Oh, how sad we all were!

We love you,
Mom

July 8, 1991

Dear Jim,

I think it's about a year ago today that we came up to the cottage—the thing you were looking forward to doing all through your bone-marrow-transplant-recovery period. It was one of your dreams—but not under these circumstances, was it?

If you hadn't had to be hooked up to the "pole" (for your TPN [total parenteral nutrition] and your antibiotics), perhaps you could have felt a bit better—as you would in the weeks to follow. But you still had a smile on your face on the picture taken at Maddens.

I feel a bit guilty telling you I was slalom water skiing just now.

My first time in three years, it took six tries—something you had been so good at and never had another chance to do. I shall always remember the many times we skied together.

I love you,
Mom

August 7, 1991

Dear Jim,

A year ago today, you had your last outing—a cookout with your friends at Bill and Helen Hutton's home. Kris Kieland picked you up and we came to bring you home. Little did we know that the following day would begin your last four days with us. Oh, how it hurts.

As I sit here in the cottage, I feel like Napoleon, abandoned on his island. The cottage is on its own moat of piers—all excavated around—as we begin to add a full basement and two room additions to the first floor. I know how difficult this coming week will be: missing you and remembering your suffering and how cheated you were. You deserved so much more for the caring, loving young man you were. You were our dream for the future and that, along with you, dear son, was taken from us. We hurt so!

Love,
Mom

August 9, 1991

Dear Jim,

It was just a year ago today that you and we were planning another trip to the cottage. But you weren't feeling too well and kept going to and from bed, thinking that very shortly we could call Dad at the office and tell him you were ready for the trip.

You finally decided against it and we called the hospice nurse in the evening. It was she who suggested we call the priest—the unspoken had now been spoken! Father Mike Krenik came out from your St. Patrick's Parish at 10:30 P.M. After he explained this was a sacrament for the sick not for the dying, you said, "Don't worry, Father, I plan on waking up tomorrow morning." Your usual good humor to bolster us all: Father Mike, Dad and Steve, Jeanne and myself. Oh, how we all miss you.

Love,
Mom

August 11, 1991

Dear Jim,

A year ago this Sunday, did you know? When you bolted up and said, "I wish, I wish . . . it doesn't matter," Dad says we asked, "What is it?" Then we laid you back on your pillow and replaced the oxygen. You never answered. Dad says it was then that you started leaving us and he prayed the rosary. After you'd spoken your last words, I believe I must have been in shock, as what immediately followed is so very vague to me. Today and yesterday, as I water-skied, an eagle flew over the lake. Was it your free spirit?

Love,
Mom

August 12, 1991

Dear Jim,

A year ago this Monday morn, on August 13, you were mercilessly taken from your once happy and promising life—and from us. So much of our happiness has gone with you. Jeanne called to see how we are doing and that means a great deal. We got through this first year on sadness and keeping busy with work. I wonder about you and life after death. You were so happy here; are you now?

I love you, dear son,
Mom

August 13, 1991

Dear Jim,

Today is the first anniversary of your death. Oh, how difficult for me to see you being taken from us. By 5:30 A.M., Dad and I realized there was no pulse in our once vibrant, loving son. Over the next four hours I sat and held your talented hands and felt them turning colder and firmer—lifeless. I had watched you perform daily at dentistry the previous four years; no other dentist will ever come near, let alone equal, your caring, thorough work. Then, at 9:30 A.M., I watched your body being carried from our home on a mortician's gurney (so much more traumatic than the many times I had sadly seen you on a hospital's surgical gurney, hooked to a myriad of tubes and monitors). I see you still, dear son, and a part of me is riveted to the last days of your life.

Later today, feeling so low (especially after watching your cousins out water skiing), I decided to go for a walk. I noticed a large bird, which I later identified as a Great Blue Heron. (I had never seen one before.) As I walked along the road, it followed me along the edge of the water. When I returned to the cottage, it was there at the shore.

When we returned home, I looked up Great Blue Heron in the phone book and found a Great Blue Heron Bookshop listed. It is across University Avenue from the Sigma Chi Fraternity House, where you'd spent many happy years. The Blue Heron is mentioned, also, in your book *Hiawatha* by Longfellow. Were you with me on this walk—present to me in spirit, to comfort? Like you, those last years, the heron didn't seem to want to pose for a picture. It would stay around until I appeared with the camera. I welcome your presence in any form.

Love,

Mom

August 15, 1991

Dear Jim,

A year ago this Thursday, on August 16—your funeral Mass! Something that shouldn't have been—but which was a beautiful tribute to you: the Sigma Chi Memorial Service and the White Rose Ceremony (which you had requested and which was executed for us by your fraternity brother, Doug Carlson); a surprise trumpet tribute by your colleague, Dr. Tom Garvin; and, then, your one-and-one-half-year-old godchild, Amanda, carrying up the Offertory gifts with the Lukens children. After the funeral luncheon, we showed your cousins, Lisa and Jim Hurtis, your beautiful office. When we got home, about ten of us went for a five-mile walk to work out some of our sadness.

Love,
Mom

August 18, 1991

Dear Jim,

This Friday, a year ago, your family gathered again for support and tore down the old deck to work out our frustrations and anger. One year later, the deck is still not finished; I am working at including some of your 1989 design plans in the finished project. You would have enjoyed the deck demolition. You and Steve always seemed to make that part of new construction your "fun forte." I even managed a hammer to my toe and, just last month (a year later), lost part of the blackened nail. I wish you were here to enjoy the "new" lake view at the cottage. Several trees have been removed for the planned walkout; you and Grandma would both have liked it.

Love,
Mom

August 25, 1991

Dear Jim,

Today, we drove to Alexandria for Tom DeWitt to replace a composite restoration that I had lost—a mesial lingual on #8! I shed tears through most of the procedure, wishing it were you doing it! This was another day of catharsis for us. Tom shared some memories of your days in Dental School: the two of you working on gold initial pendants for Linda and me in 1983; your drive home together from a Sigma Chi party; and your smudged face on gold-bridge-assignment day. The pièce de resistance: he shared with us their staged photo of your telling a story to your dental peers, during which they all doze off. You always were the great communicator who loved to share a story! We cried again, as Tom said *he* had done on his two-hour drive back to Alexandria after your wake.

We think we shall be having our future dental appointments in Alexandria with the dentist you chose to do your own dental work. First, however, we shall support Regina, the dentist who bought your practice, for a few years more.

Love to you, Dr. Jim,
Mom

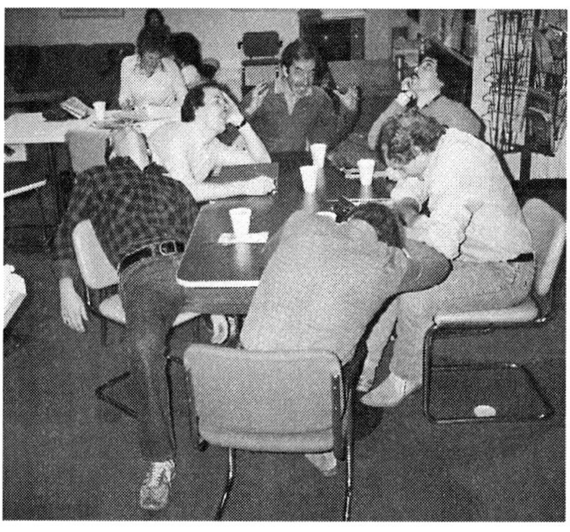

The "staged" photo.
August 25, 1991
(Photo courtesy of
Dr. Tom DeWitt)

August 28, 1991

Dear Jim,

A year ago (about a week after your funeral), Dad was told by Fina Oil Company, that it was his last day. He was being "let go because his productivity has been down the past month," they said—in spite of the fact that he had gone into the office each of your last days with us. His days could have been spent with you. What a slap in the face, and what a lousy way to replace someone when the truth would not have been so heartless. Being told he was being replaced by someone younger and less expensive on their payroll would have been so much easier to accept.

With regrets for you and Dad,
Mom

September 5, 1991

Dear Jim,

Janssens came up to the cottage today—the first time since you died. Ron went down to the dock and spent some time with his thoughts about you and about seeing you here at the anniversary last year. At dinner we reminisced—including the story Ron told of how he brought you in from water skiing (the time you skied almost to shore) and he was so afraid you would hit land. We remembered, too, your favorite family incident—Dad and Ron's attempt to free the "shored" pontoon boat. Joan told of your visits to the Arboretum last year when she picked you up from the hospital for daytime passes. We all cried. You could expect that of Grandpa and me—but Dad and Ron?

Were you with us in spirit, as you were in our days of joy?

Love,
Mom

October 6, 1991

Jim, dear son,

Remember the fire that burns for you in my heart as I plod onward!

Love,
Mom

October 11, 1991

Dear Jim,

Today is the first anniversary of your grandmother's death. Though I miss her, I know you are together in heaven. I feel I never fully grieved Grandma's death because it came less than two months after you were taken from us; I was still in such intense grief over our loss of you. I think perhaps she was more deeply affected by your death than we realized; and she must have been tired. She had had a long and happy life. But I never thought, as I visited her in the hospital, that she would not be discharged soon from her broken hip. Are you and she speaking in German as you sometimes did in fun?

Love,
Mom

October 17, 1991

Dear Jim,

It's three years ago today (in 1988, the year that your practice had grown and you would pay off your loans and investment), as I sat typing letters for one of our marketing lists, that I received your concerned phone call asking me to meet you at the University of Minnesota Hospital. You had been called at the clinic and told something had shown up on the CAT scan. Though you had been told the week before that the scan was fine, they had forgotten to read the second. As surgery was being scheduled for the following day, it was a sad wait we had in Admissions. You were both frightened and dejected and I felt so helpless. Life can change so in one day. Just the day previous, we'd had a happy day—a baby shower for your sister, Jeanne.

Those marketing letters were never sent. We did not know, then, that your promising career and a long and happy life were never to be realized.

Yesterday Dad and I brought a large boulder to a treed area at the cottage for what will one day be a meditation area.

We love you,
Mom

November 22, 1991

Dear Jim,

"Mom, I may die."

Two years ago you spoke those terrible words to me—across the reception desk at your dental practice. You had been to see your oncologist at the U of M that day and she gave you the harsh news. She had said she thought I'd be with you at your appointment; never had she indicated that something of this magnitude would be discussed! What a terrible thing to be told; how heartless to tell someone alone!

From Day One, in December of 1985, I felt she never showed you any true compassion or caring. She never visited you in the hospital, though she ordered the admissions for surgery and tests so many times in the four years she was your doctor. Dr. Longo at the University of Wisconsin Hospital was most caring and compassionate and visited you each day.

As we left work that awful day, you waved good-bye as usual. But I would never see that self-confident grin again. Yet the memory of it remains etched in my mind.

Love,
Mom

January 3, 1992

Dear Jim,

It was two years ago, while I sat with you following your bone marrow harvest and first series of high-dose chemotherapy (in Madison, at the University of Wisconsin Hospital), that you expressed your feelings regarding the awful sentence given you. It was the only time in all of your suffering that you had done so. "Why must I suffer so? Am I so different from my brothers and sisters?" How does a mother answer such a fine, gentle, loving son who deserved so much more, who never gave us one instance of concern, who had worked so hard for the success he would achieve and then not live to enjoy. I shall never understand!

Love,
Mom

January 15, 1992

Dear Jim,

Two years have passed since you saw your last dental patient. You were feeling lousy and, while waiting for some dental x-rays to process, had lain down to rest in the unused dental chair. You would subsequently be hospitalized at the U of M for one of the many infections that followed your monthly rounds of high-dose chemo in Madison. This was all to have been a part of the cure—but less debilitating, we thought. I miss you and I hurt for you.

Love,
Mom

April 5, 1992

Dear Jim,

Your birthdate—once a happy day for me! On your 32nd, your last birthday two years ago, you and I spent the day in your hospital room in the bone marrow transplant unit at the University of Wisconsin. Hardly a happy day for you! The nurses brought in a bottle of champagne, which we weren't allowed to open, of course. Joan Janssen brought an inflatable birthday cake and we sang (all with masks, gowns, gloves and booties).

It was just a week after your bone marrow transplant and you were progressing well—according to all projections. Though you couldn't eat or drink, we celebrated by concentrating on your gifts: a jacket from your brother, Steve; a journal from your sister, Jeanne; a portable CD player from Dad and me.

How I wish we could all be reminiscing with you about this unusual birthday. Steve and Amanda will be with Dad and me for a dinner of some of your favorite foods: ham, sweet potatoes, and Nana's strawberry torte.

I love and miss you and wish you would still be bounding up the steps, two at a time, calling out, "Mom, I'm home." I can't believe I am having trouble recalling your voice and am looking for some tapes or videos on which we might hear it once again.

Love,
Mom

May 17, 1992

Dear Jim,

Once again, I am writing on the 17th of May. Today could have been perfect. Had you been here, it could have been a real party! It was, instead, a gathering of about sixty of your family and friends: Hill-Murray, Sigma Chi, and DDS. Bryan came from Michigan to join the rest of your family. As you requested, we had the party to use the $400 your Hill-Murray and Card Club friends gave you in July of 1990. You had entreated them to take it back. When they would not, you asked me (if you did not make it) to use it for this purpose. In addition, we decided to give them something in your memory. So, we presented to each of the card club couples two Jackson & Perkins Simplicity rose bushes—the kind of rose you grew at your home in Edina. I believe it was Kathy's idea that we give these and they all were most happy with them. The newly finished deck includes some of your design and the raised planter surrounding it has, for us, reminders of your landscaping: the Simplicity roses, with Alberta spruce at each end and a corkscrew willow below.

You would have had a ball. As it is, your spirit was here in all your glory—present in the exceptional friends you had chosen in your life! Per your specifications, we had volleyball, beer and ham. Per my request, everyone shared a memento of you: written thoughts, a video tape with you and your voice, pictures, and a poem you had written—in *your* writing. Woody Larson had dug through boxes until he found it!

I must write this before I read the reminiscences; I shall be too teary-eyed after. It was a bittersweet day.

Love,

Mom

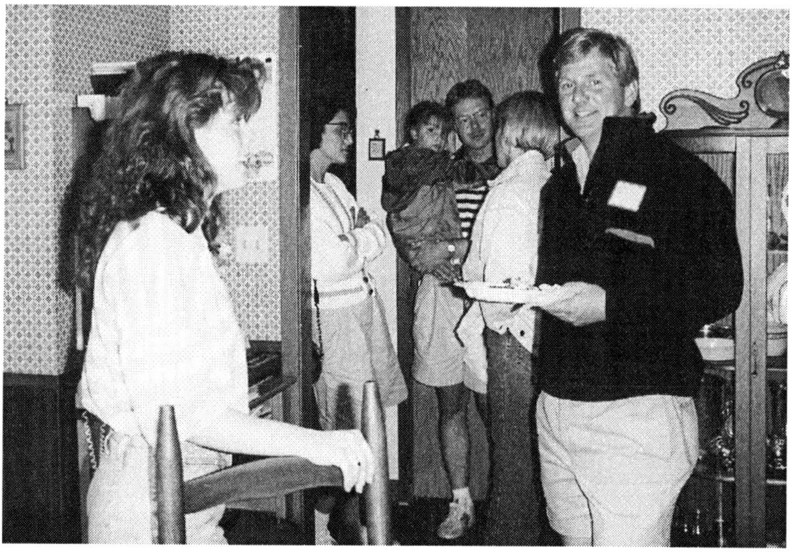

Shelly Kraimer; Mary, Lisa and John Poppenberg; Terry McNeice Larson; Woody Larson

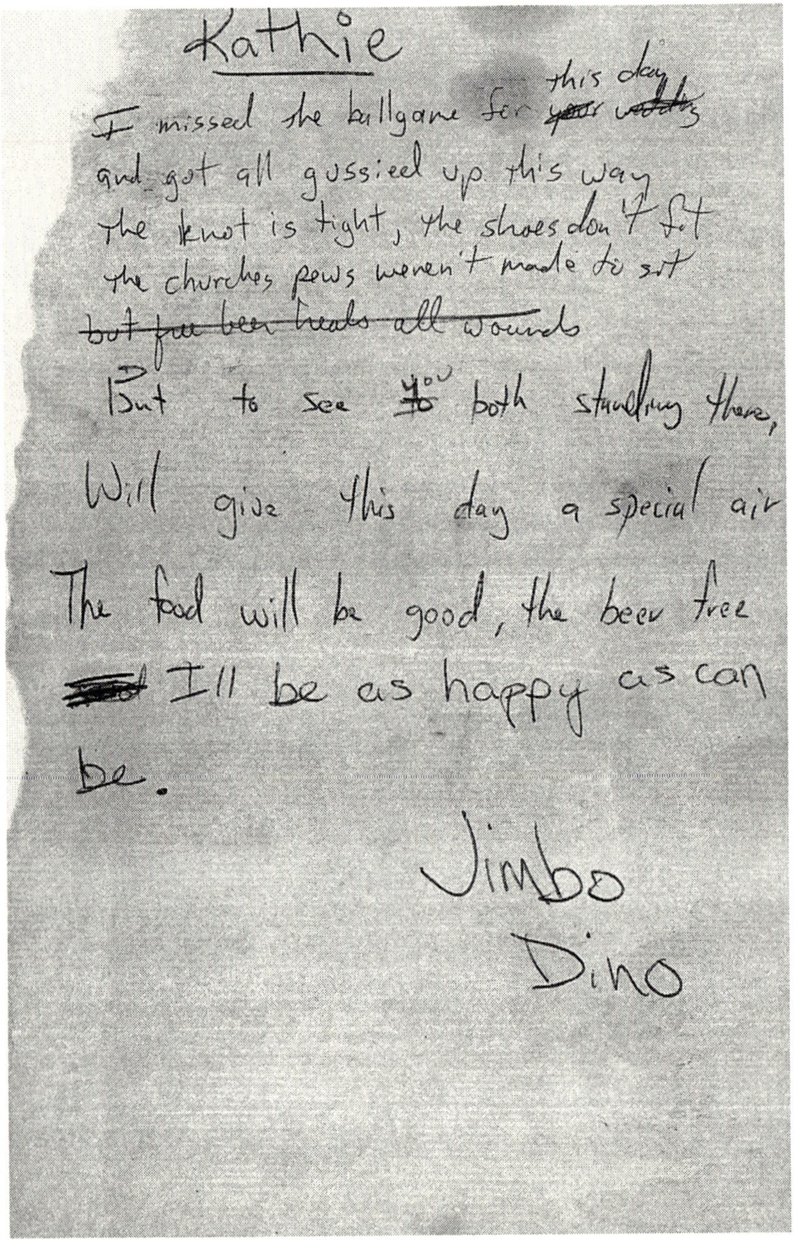

Kathie

I missed the ballgame for ~~your wedding~~ this day
and got all gussied up this way
The knot is tight, the shoes don't fit
the churches pews weren't made to sit
~~but free beer heals all~~ wounds

But to see ~~to~~ you both standing there,
Will give this day a special air
The food will be good, the beer free
~~And~~ I'll be as happy as can
be.

Jimbo
Dino

Jim's Sigma Chi friend, Woody Larson, found this poem, in Jim's handwriting, on the original paper. It was penned for the bride of Tim Meehan, a fraternity brother.

May 18, 1992

Dear Jim,

Last night I read all of the reminiscences that your friends, doctors, colleagues, and patients brought or sent to yesterday's party. I know you will have to bear with me as I recount them; but I must. Repeatedly used were the adjectives kind and good; happy and carefree; cheerful and optimistic; patient, especially with children; courageous and brave. Attributes included a strong spirit; of gentle ways; hard-working and of good morals; intensity for life; a gentle charm; loved philosophical discussions; and, a person harboring a big secret about the best that life has to offer. Descriptions of you as beautiful, with sparkling blue eyes; gentle and kind eyes; shy, sweet smiling face. I know this reads like a litany but these were all well-earned accolades. You would be embarrassed, I know.

You are worth every tear I shed,
Mom

July 25, 1992

Dear Jim,

Today we returned from our trip to the Northwest in order to be home for your grandfather's 90th birthday. Before we left, I called Eileen to find out the places where you had gone with Brad, Eileen, and Terry in 1985. Though we didn't backpack or fish, we wanted to "walk your walk." We saw the places where you had been: the Badlands, Mount Rushmore, Devils Tower, the Bighorn Mountains, and Beartooth Highway. It felt good. Then, we went on to Glacier, Washington, and Oregon. I am so happy that, as a family, we had seen all but sixteen states together.

Love,
Mom

August 13, 1992

Dear Jim,

Again this year we find ourselves at the cottage. The most difficult time for me is the day and evening before the anniversary of your death as I find I relive and feel the pain of each minute. After last year, I also realize that I must be in control of our surroundings on these days. In order to be alone with our thoughts of you, Dad and I went for a 10-mile walk on Bearskin Trail. A beautiful butterfly appeared and made the walk with us; we felt your presence.

Then we joined Father Abts for a private Mass—said for you. Jeanne called again on this anniversary to share our sorrow.

You are remembered always,
Mom

September 3, 1992

Dear Jim,

Today we received a letter from Long Island, NY—from a Gloria Fremed, someone we did not know. She belongs to a Long Island Chapter of Compassionate Friends. Our Hudson Chapter, along with other chapters, had made and sent *butterflies* to the National Conference of Compassionate Friends. Gloria selected ours and, on reading our attached information as she walked away, knew her selection of our *butterfly* was not happenstance.

Like us, she has lost a son to cancer. Like you, Clifford was a dentist. Like you, he died at age 32. Gloria believed a greater power had directed her to our *butterfly*. She described her son as a caretaker, an exceptional young man with an unbelievable smile—qualities everyone remembers in you.

I will be writing to Gloria telling her of *our* skillful dentist and gentle, loving son whom we miss so very much.

Love,
Mom

December 20, 1992

Dear Jim,

Today as I was reading one of your favorite comic strips, *B.C.*, I found this—a message from you? It shall make my Christmas a bit brighter.

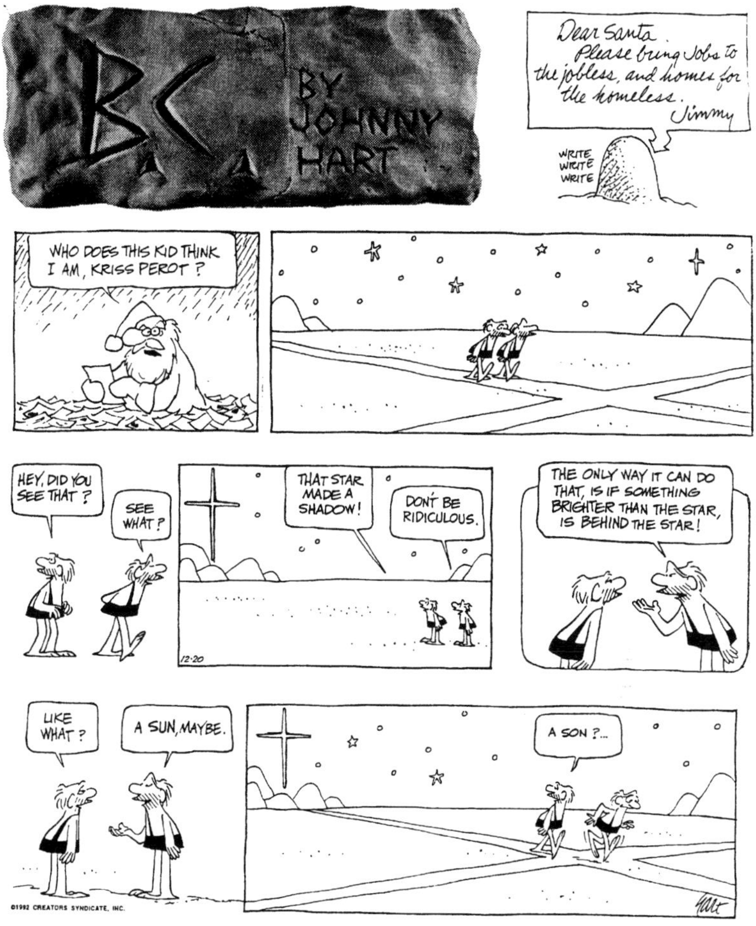

BC
BY JOHNNY HART
Dear Santa. Please bring Jobs to the jobless, and homes for the homeless. Jimmy
WRITE WRITE WRITE
WHO DOES THIS KID THINK I AM, KRISS PEROT ?
HEY, DID YOU SEE THAT ?
SEE WHAT ?
THAT STAR MADE A SHADOW !
DON'T BE RIDICULOUS.
12·20
THE ONLY WAY IT CAN DO THAT, IS IF SOMETHING BRIGHTER THAN THE STAR, IS BEHIND THE STAR !
LIKE WHAT ?
A SUN, MAYBE.
A SON ?...
©1992 CREATORS SYNDICATE, INC.

"By permission of Johnny Hart and Creators Syndicate, Inc."

Merry Christmas, Jim
Mom

April 10, 1993—Holy Saturday

Dear Jim,

We now have a portrait of you in our living room!

A dear high-school friend of mine, Vivian Kukulka Krieg, took up painting after the death of her daughter, Anne. Though she had never done a portrait before, Vivian agreed to do one of you. She worked against some rules: she had to paint from a photo, and I wanted you smiling. She requested various other photos of you, and we spoke of you at length. As Vivian had not known you, she asked that we send anything we had that might enable her to know you. One of the things we sent was a copy of your will. On reading it, her husband, George, decided to add to his will your request that beneficiaries donate 10 percent of their inheritance to their favorite charities.

Vivian is a compassionate and gifted artist. The painting is beautiful and we now have the spirit of you ever present with us.

When I told Vivian of our Great Blue Heron experience, she told me she really believes our deceased children choose ways to communicate with us.

Love is eternal,
Mom

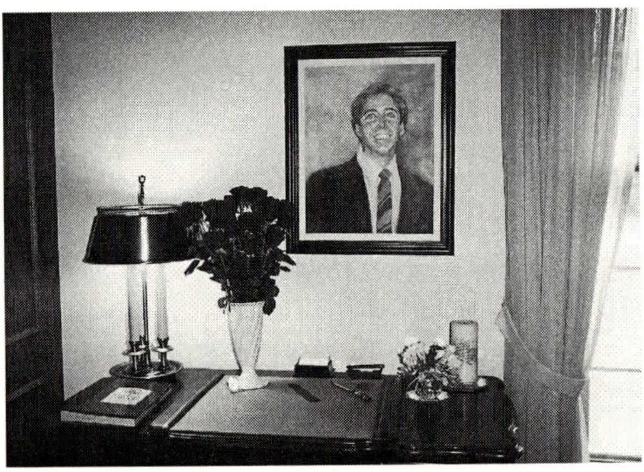

April 10, 1993

June 15, 1993

Dear Jim,

I'm frightened! Today, at my annual gynecology appointment, Dr. Spraitz found another lump in my abdominal area. Another laparotomy is being scheduled. I feel more scared now than I did in 1990. Is it because, then, you were still with me? As I lay on the table for my ultrasound, I could not stop shaking.

Is this why you appeared to me in my dream? You said, "Mom, I'm happy, I'm really happy." I was so thankful for this short dream. Previously, all my dreams of you have been of your suffering, and your presence is always accompanied by my thought, "Jim, though not yet well, is still with us." This dream meant so much to me. Hearing your voice in person would be so much better, but I will have to settle for this. Thank you!

Love,

Mom

"If someone you've cared about has died, perhaps you've wondered about the fact that you don't seem to dream about them very often. I would expect that a loss would trigger subconscious thoughts that would find expression in dreams. I am now convinced that the number of times you dream about that person is not important. What matters is that when it does happen, you get a message that will help you continue to live with acceptance of what cannot be changed."

—Rosita Perez, *The Music is You*

Sept. 28, 1994

Dear Jim,

Today we returned to your fraternity, Sigma Chi, for a bittersweet evening—the dedication for the restoration of the stained glass window. This was a tribute to you and a celebration of your life. Per your request in your will (that your beneficiaries donate 10 percent of their inheritance to charity), we chose as one of our bequests a gift to Sigma Chi (ΣX), where you'd spent happy years and made some lifelong friends.

Being there brought back memories of our many visits when you were a student at the university and I was president of the ΣX Mothers' Club—Curry Dinners and Sweetheart Teas. We were

The Brother

James J. Deininger D.D.S

Dedication

Sigma Chi Fraternity

September 28, 1994

7:00 - 8:00 PM

Social	***Hosted by Helen Peterson***
Welcoming and Introductions; Opening thoughts and purpose	***Bret Lathrop***
Music	***Mike Pretasky***
Presentation of the plaque	***Bret Lathrop***
Sigma Chi Ritually acknowledged dedication	***Doug Carlson***
Social	

"All honor to his name"

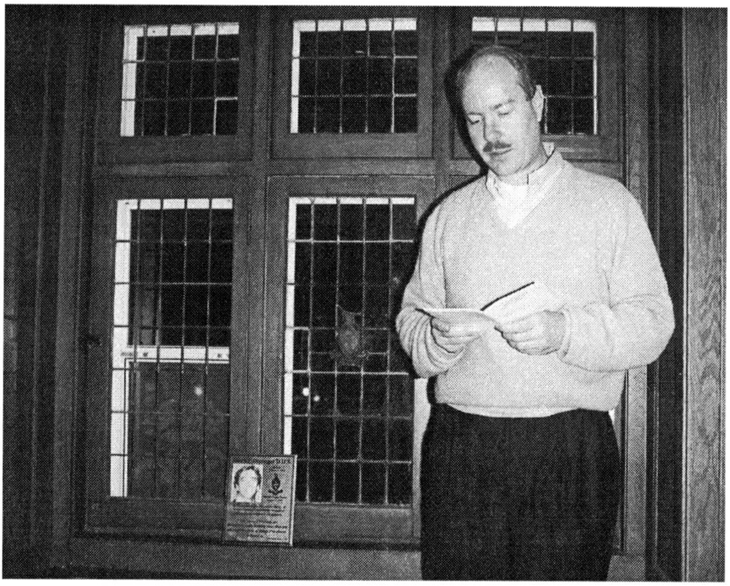

Doug Carlson, fraternity brother, who worked on this fitting tribute to Jim

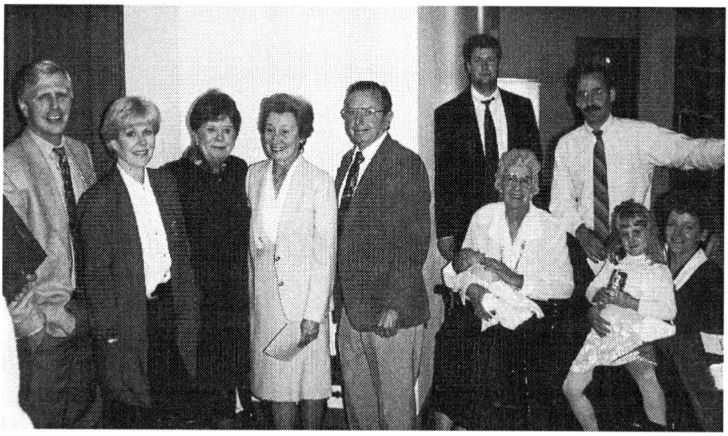

Fraternity brother, Randy Larson, and wife Terry; parent, Mary Bornhofen; Dona and Al; fraternity brother, John Yung; housemother, Helen Peterson, holding sister Jeanne's son, Ryan; brother and fraternity brother, Steve; Amanda, daughter of Jeanne, and Jeanne

always so proud of you and enjoyed meeting and making friends with the parents of your frat brothers. Many of them were there: Doug Carlson (who helped us find a fitting memorial in your honor, then execute the plaque and dedication ceremony); Terry and Randy Larson, John Yung and his parents, Georgianne and Ray Yung; Mary Bornhofen, the ΣX residents and housemother; and Steve, Jeanne, Amanda, and three-week-old, Ryan.

The window is beautifully restored; and, as a fitting tribute to you, Sigma Chi had a plaque done. It has an engraved picture of you and a quote we chose from your Indoctrination letter to us: "The Sigma Chi ideals are themselves really nothing new; they are all reaffirmations of things I've always believed in."

Honored and drained,
Mom

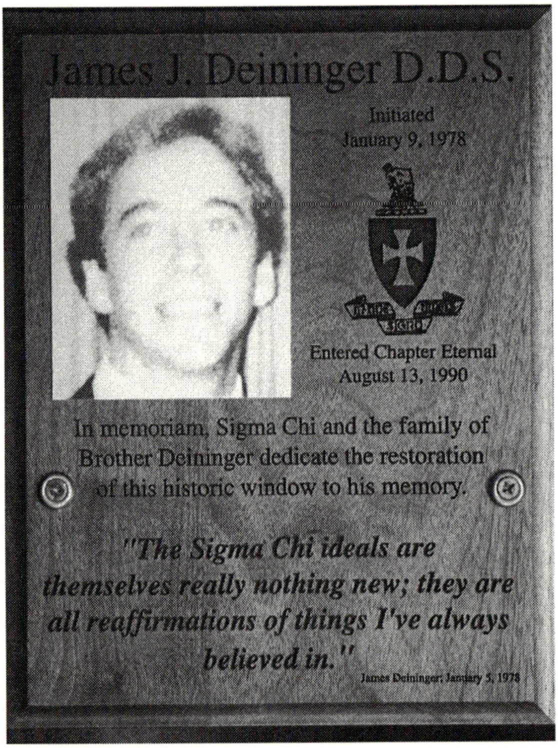

November 1, 1994

Dear Jim,

All Saints' Day—a day to remember our special saint in Heaven, you! Dad and I went to Mass this morning and I could only remember that five years ago you and I had gone to noon Mass together at St. Patrick's (during our lunch break at your practice).

Those were days of apprehension as we went to daily Mass. We were concerned because your oncologist had noted your elevated monocyte count and you were experiencing a cough that seemed to be like the one you'd had in the summer of 1988—an ominous note for us as we prayed and hoped.

Love,

Mom

November 2, 1994

Dear Jim,

We just returned from an All Souls' Day Remembrance Service at St. Mary's Church. In years past, we would go to Mass on this day to remember the deceased souls in our family—our grandparents. Never did I think we would some day be doing so for one of our children.

Five years ago, we were all together celebrating your godchild Amanda's first birthday—joyous and happy that your chemo was behind you. Now we could put our lives back together, we thought!

We didn't, did we?

Love,

Mom

July 29, 1995

Dear Jim,

Yesterday we returned home from the funeral of your grandfather; he died the day before we were going to Wausau for his 93rd birthday. I regret so much that no one called to inform me that he was not doing well that day. Would you please tell him I am so sorry that I could not visit him one more time and hear him say, "Oh, Dona Mae, you're here." Now all of your grandparents are with you; you're there much too early!

Today we were invited by Jim and Kathy Miettunen to attend the dedication of the new brick entry to St. Joseph's Home for Children in Minneapolis. After your death, they had chosen to give to this charity in your memory; and they have done so on occasions such as Christmas and the anniversaries of your birth and death. Now they have donated one of the tiles, engraved with your name. Another tribute to our son whom we miss so much!

Love,

Mom

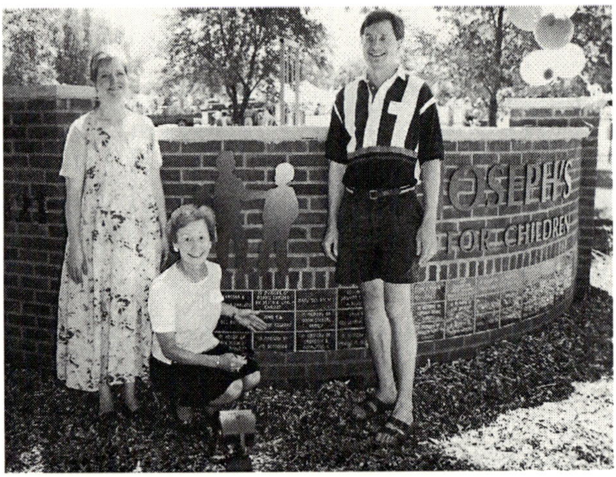

With Cathy and Jim Miettunen at dedication of brick entry wall at St. Joseph's Home for Children—1121 E. 46th St., Minneapolis, Minnesota

Granite tile within brick entry wall

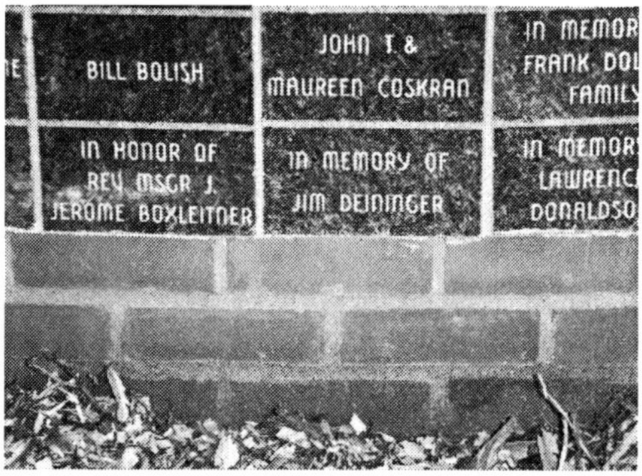
BILL BOLISH
JOHN T &
MAUREEN COSKRAN
IN HONOR OF
REV MSGR J.
JEROME BOXLEITNER
IN MEMORY OF
JIM DEININGER

January 1, 1996

Dear Jim,

Today we returned from our first New Year's Eve weekend spent at the cottage. It was Jeanne's idea and you would have enjoyed it! How I wish we had done that for one of the New Year's Eves when you were with us. You liked outdoor fun (especially on Thanksgiving and New Year's Eve). We saucer-sledded down the cottage hill with Amanda and Ryan, and Dad "luged" the sides. I resurrected the game of "pie" and we introduced it to Amanda.

Love,
Mom

January 8, 1996

Dear Jim,

This day I took a 5-mile walk, going through Pine Tree Estates. I saw the footbridges on the ends of Pine Tree Lake and remembered our cross-country ski jaunts together. One time we were gone so long that Dad and Steve wondered where we were and whether I had forgotten the roast I had put in the oven before we left. No more shared experiences with you. I have only memories, and though they are all great ones, I am sad and lost.

Your XC skiing partner,
Mom

April 6, 1996

Dear Jim,

On this Holy Saturday, the day after your birthdate, Steve's fiancée, Marsha, was baptized and received into our Catholic faith. We were so proud of and happy for them both, and I know you must be, too. Because you were born on Holy Saturday, it was very symbolic for me. I remember how proud and happy we were 38 years ago.

Love,

Mom

August 23, 1996 - Steve & Marsha's wedding

Dear Jim,

"This was a fun party," Amanda said. And it truly was. Two-year-old Ryan performed his duties as ring bearer wonderfully; having Amanda walk next to him as a flower girl helped. Everyone commented on the beautiful wedding and reception. You would have had a great time with us! We are all so very happy for Steve and Marsha. The picture of our surviving family turned out so well; we are missing only your handsome presence.

Love,

Mom

Thanksgiving 1996

Dear Jim,

Today, as the family gathered, Marsha commented that she had seen Dr. Haas, the oral surgeon you knew and to whom you made referrals. Noticing Marsha's last name, he asked if she might be related to you, and, on hearing she was, he spoke of you and what a wonderful dentist you were. We wish you were still—with us and available to us as our dentist.

Marsha has made me feel so very good. Through all of her decisions for dentistry work—a diastema, extractions, braces—she always asks my opinion regarding both the proposed procedures and the referrals. It has given me a chance to use the knowledge and terms you taught me.

Love,

Mom

April 27, 1997

Dear Jim,

Today your godchild, Amanda, made her First Communion. I wish you could have been here to celebrate with her. You should have been allowed that. Her godmother never comes. In your absence, I'm happy for dear Amanda that Steve and Marsha step in to act as proxy godparents for her.

At the Communion Mass, we sat in front of Kathy Mishek, whose daughter also made her First Communion. Kathy remembered you and had not known you had died. Do you remember how thankful we were when you were not seriously injured in the car accident in which you were broadsided and the Vega was "totaled"? We remember, too, when you were living at the fraternity house at the time of the "great fire." Sigma Chi just had another, less extensive fire.

Had you been with us today, all five siblings would have been present.

Love,

Mom

December 6, 1997

Dear Jim,

On this feast day of St. Nicholas, as I was walking out of Kowalski's grocery store, I heard two young Boy Scouts singing, and I immediately thought of you. You would have appreciated their young entrepreneurial skills. They were selling Christmas wreaths, as you once did in Madison. To bolster sales (and in the Christmas spirit), they were singing to the melody of *Oh, Christmas Tree,* words that went something like this: "Oh, Christmas wreath, Oh, Christmas wreath; They're only seven dollars."

Grinning, remembering, and sad, I thought of you.
Mom

January 22, 1998

Dear Jim,

As I await a breast biopsy tomorrow, I realize how much of my strength was in you. I remember the days before and after my laparatomy in 1990, when I was diagnosed with colon cancer and given a 40–45 percent prognosis! It seems I got through those difficult times less frightened than I am now. And so, my dear son and special saint in heaven, I ask your prayers and intercession for me now as I approach this surgery—that the suspicious and indeterminate breast calcifications will be benign.

I love you and give thanks for you,
Mom

February 10, 1998

Dear Jim,

Today we found ourselves driving into the parking lot at the University of Wisconsin Clinic. It was the first time we had done so since July 1990, when we arrived for your discharge. That was done with heavy hearts, after you had been told you had weeks to live. Now it brought a flood of emotions and tears.

This time, it is for me to see a breast-cancer surgeon for these suspicious calcifications. Again, I ask your prayers for me—that his opinion will be a favorable one.

Love,

Mom

April 5, 1998

Dear Jim,

Today your family and friends met to remember you on your 40th birthday. How I wish that you could have been with us and that your friends could have been teasing you about being "over the hill." Instead, we received their support and compassion.

Jeanne, Steve and Bryan were able to be here, though Kathy wasn't. And the Miettunens, Helen Hutton, and Mike Rieschl and sons joined us at 7:30 Mass. Father Bill had the Mass and joined us at the house later. To all of your family and friends, Dad and I presented packets of notes we had had printed, with your painting of *Dad in Denims* on the front. Mike remembered when you painted it in the art class you took together.

During a ham brunch, we viewed a new video, transferred from our home movies. It goes from your birth to that of Bryan's. Our dear friends Dee and Frankie Marks joined us and became more acquainted with you—as a toddler, that is. We had some good laughs, remembering the baby chicks from Schaibles and how your chick, "Doc," managed to survive as the two of you became acquainted!

The Larson family could not come but Mike Yung came, and we had a good day reminiscing and sharing our loss.

You certainly knew how to choose good friends.

Happy Birthday and Love,

Mom

August 22, 1998—Jeanne and Bill's wedding

Dear Jim,

Two years after Steve and Marsha's wedding, your family gathered for another. Jeanne, Amanda, and Ryan walked up the aisle on this day to marry Bill. We are most happy for all of them. We welcome Bill, who has never been married and who is so happy to gain both a wife and a family in one day. The ceremony was beautiful and the reception and dinner were large. So many of your cousins came and were excited about being together again. Bill, knowing how much I missed your presence, was thoughtful in speaking of you at the dinner.

Love,

Mom

February 2, 1999

Dear Jim,

Today, at the University of Wisconsin clinic, I was told I could return to annual mammograms. I thank you again for your intercessions on my behalf. You continue to be my special guardian angel and "the wind beneath my wings."

Love,

Mom

April 3, 1999—Holy Saturday

Dear Jim,

This is another anniversary of the religious holiday on which you were born. Forty-one years ago we welcomed you into the world; today we welcomed Jeanne's husband, Bill, into our Catholic faith—just as we welcomed Marsha three years ago. I find this all very significant. Are you rejoicing with us?

Love,

Mom

July 7, 1999

Dear Jim,

Today we returned home from the cottage after I was discharged yesterday from Wausau Hospital. I had a heart attack last Friday at the cottage, shortly after going three-generation-skiing with Jeanne and Amanda. Are you as shocked as your family, my doctors, and I? Given no risk factors, my health-care professionals suggest it may have been stress. Could it be the letter I received which threatens to sever the family ties from my only sibling? Now I begin six weeks of cardiac rehabilitation. I pray for acceptance of this rebuff, for my emotions to heal, and for healing in our family.

In spending the Fourth of July in the hospital, I missed the Deininger Cousins' Reunion—as did you. I had had special T-shirts done for all of our family. Each had a different picture of you with the person wearing the shirt. I *hope* you didn't mind! However, I didn't get to wear mine—nor did Bryan. His shirt was locked in one of the cars—along with the car keys. Bryan and I shall wear our new shirts at another gathering. I also had note cards made for all your cousins and aunts. The face of the card was your oil painting of *Dad in Denims.*

Love,

Mom

June 16, 2000—Friday

Dear Jim,

With this entry, I shall complete this journal and move to publication. Today Dad and I observed our Golden Wedding Anniversary. I know you would have been so happy to celebrate with us. The only way I could justify a celebration was to include you in the liturgy and festivities. I hope you approved of your portrait being in the sanctuary of the church for Mass; it was meant to be a reminder of the fact that you are with us still.

Father Mike, now the pastor at St. Pius X, was happy to be with us for the day, and we appreciated his presence and his remembering. The soloist, a beautiful tenor (as you were), and the pianist reminded me of the days when, at the U, you took voice lessons, and you and I would practice our singing and piano skills late at night. Your godchild, Amanda, read the petitions so well, including those for you and your four grandparents. Marsha, Gary, and Bill did the readings. Do you remember when you and your siblings gave us silver bands on our 25th anniversary and presented them with the remark, "When you are married 50 years, you'll get the gold." Promise kept! Today, at the Mass, your brothers and sisters presented us with the gold bands. It was a beautiful day; you would have enjoyed being present in more than spirit, I know. You would have appreciated the wonderful luncheon. And wasn't the happiness of family and friends a joy to see?

Love and Auf Wiedersehen,
Mom

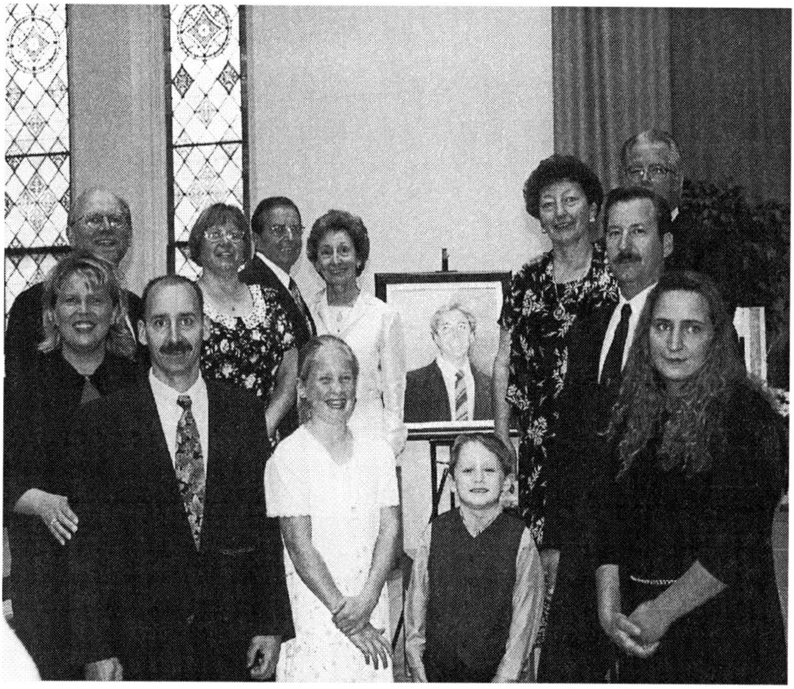

Our family that was able to be present at our Golden Anniversary Mass. Clockwise, beginning in front of Jim's portrait: Ryan, our grandson; Amanda, our granddaughter; our son, Steve; our daughter-in-law, Marsha; our son-in-law, Bill Hartman; our daughter, Jeanne; Al and myself. To the right of our son Jim's portrait: our daughter, Kathy Lukens; our son-in-law, Gary; our son, Bryan, and our granddaughter, Terri Lukens.

Afterword

THROUGHOUT THIS JOURNEY WITHOUT JIM, WE ARE MOST thankful for our family and friends who have journeyed with us. Jim's friends from Hill-Murray High School and Sigma Chi fraternity have called, visited, and written us often. Our own friends, too, have realized our need for company and socialization. For example, shortly after Jim's funeral, and before Kathy and her family returned home, my cousins Glenn and Ursula invited all of us for an evening cruise on their boat. Some time later they entertained only Al and me for a quiet Sunday. Only later did they invite us to share an evening with added guests. It was this thoughtfulness by so many of our friends that allowed us to gradually reenter society. One day, years after we'd given the rose bushes from the money Jim's Hill-Murray friends had given him, we received a letter and photo from April and Dave Paddock. When one of their moves from state to state was going to take place in the winter, in order to keep the roses, they had transplanted them in the fall to the home of relatives.

Grief and support groups have also been helpful for us on this unplanned journey. The week after Jim's death, Bruce Kuritsky of St. Joseph's Hospice came out to our home to give our family insights into the grief journey ahead of us. This personal presentation was most helpful to those of us who could be here—our children, Jeanne and Steve, our granddaughter Terri, Al and me. The following month, Al and I, along with Steve and Jeanne, attended a grief support session at Jim's parish, St. Patrick in Edina. I often worried about Kathy and Bryan who lived at a distance and could not be with us at the grief and support sessions.

During September, October, and November of 1990, we attended a series of seven weekly sessions on Growing through Loss, offered by Trinity Lutheran Church in Stillwater. These were especially helpful because, after the general presentation, we broke into individual groups: Loss of Child (for Al and me), and Loss of Sibling (for Jeanne). When my father spent some time with us after my mother's death, he took part in the Loss of Spouse group. At this time, had the individual groups not all met simultaneously, Al and I would have qualified for three: Loss of Child, Loss of Parent, and Loss of Job. Then in February, March and April, we attended a six-session education and support group program at the Hospice of HealthEast—St. Joseph's Hospital. Jeanne also accompanied us to these.

In November of 1991, we attended our first meeting of The Compassionate Friends—St. Croix Valley Chapter, in Hudson, Wisconsin. The Compassionate Friends, founded in England in 1969 by a hospital chaplain, is a self-help organization offering friendship and understanding to bereaved parents. In the mutual grieving of two parent-couples, they discovered that by listening to one another, by crying together when they felt like doing so, by understanding how each felt, the bereaved parents grief was lessened. This then became an international organization.

For the first years, I was unable to get through sharing our story at introductions to a group. Only a few broken and choked words came from me, tears ran down my face and I couldn't go on. Al had to handle that introductory sharing for both of us. Now I do better. Al and I have experienced much sharing and caring in this group—for everyone knows and understands the pain. We continue our journey with them and help in facilitating at some of the monthly meetings.

I have, also, in the past few years been involved in the bereavement ministry program at our parish, St. Mary of the Lake. There are presently nine of us who have been trained in this ministry. As a Bereavement Minister I visit individually with parishioners up to eighteen months after the death of a loved one. It is a time of compassionate presence and listening as the bereaved travel the grieving journey.

To share our own loss, at one of our Thanksgiving family gatherings, I asked everyone to give their favorite memory of Jim or express how they missed him most. Al remembered a frantic call from Jim to change the dental cabinets when he noticed a discrepancy of inches in the floor plan at the office. Steve said he missed doing things with Jim. In working together on various projects, they would call Al for help and, invariably, end up messing up Dad's organization of tools. Bryan remembered Boy Scouts and some advice Jim gave him before one of his campouts. "Soap the pan before cooking," Jim said. Not specifying, "Soap only the outside," the result was soapy pancakes! Jeanne remembers the get-togethers with laughing, singing and playing guitars and she misses Jim the most when she thinks about the void in our lives with him being gone. Kathy misses his telling stories to the kids and the times they spent together when he was with them in Madison. Terri missed coming home from school and being able to talk and watch television together. And my father, Jim's grandfather, said, "Jim was always close to Grandma."

Our four surviving children continue to bring joy and meaning to our lives. When we are all together I delight in watching their interaction with each other. I only wish Jim were present to add to the repartee. Keeping busy and spending time with our children and our grandchildren help fill our days and years. I try to use my gift of life to the utmost for I realize how precious each day is and how fragile life is.